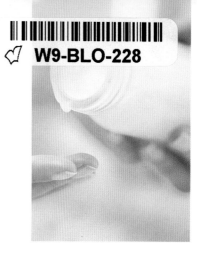

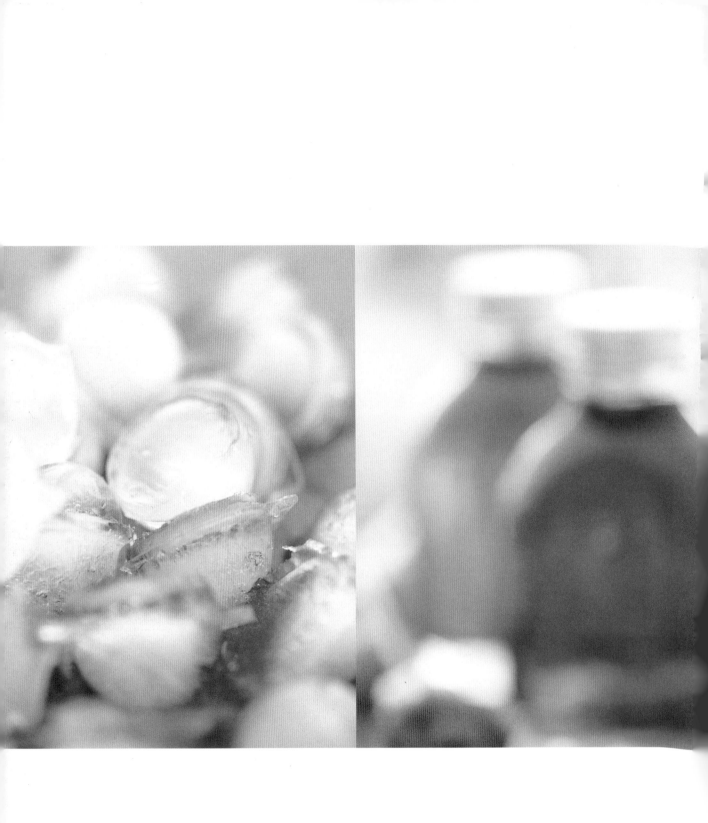

home health spa

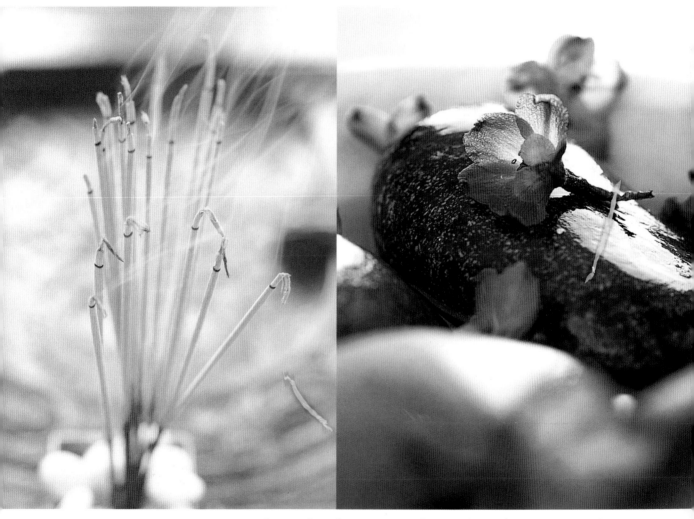

weekend plans to detox, relax & energize

anna selby

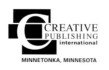

CREATIVE PUBLISHING international

MINNETONKA, MINNESOTA

www.howtobookstore.com

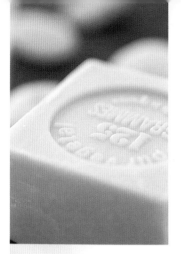
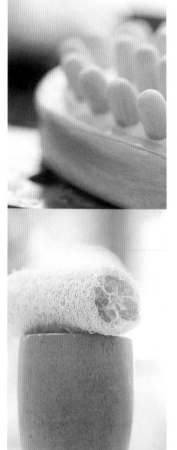
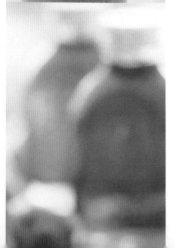

First published in the USA and Canada in 2001 by
Creative Publishing international, Inc.

CREATIVE
PUBLISHING
international

President/CEO David D. Murphy
Vice President/Editorial Patricia K. Jacobsen
Vice President/Retail Sales and Marketing Richard M. Miller
Executive Editor/Lifestyles Department Elaine Perry

First published in Great Britain in 2000 by Hamlyn, a division of
Octopus Publishing Group Limited
2–4 Heron Quays, London, E14 4JP

Copyright © 2000 Octopus Publishing Group Limited

Publishing Director Alison Goff
Executive Editor Jane McIntosh
Project Editor Katey Day
Copy Editor Casey Horton
Creative Director Keith Martin
Design Manager Bryan Dunn
Senior Designer Claire Harvey
Special Photography Ian Wallace
Stylist Clare Hunt
Models Chantal Johansson at M&P Management plc and
   Malin Johansson at M&P Management plc
Picture Researchers Christine Junemann and Rosie Garai
Production Controller Lisa Moore

ISBN 0-86573-148-9

Printed in Hong Kong
10 9 8 7 6 5 4 3 2 1

All special photography by Ian Wallace
Except for Octopus Publishing Group Ltd./Jean Cazals 95/Graham Kirk 14,
15, 38, 39, 40, 73, 74/Sandra Lane 21, 52, 53/Gary Latham 104,
105/William Adams-Lingwood 23, 35/David Loftus 20/Diana Miller 54,
94/Peter Myers 13, 55, 72, 75, 97/Bill Reavell 67 Top, 67 Bottom/Paul
Williams 66

Recipe Notes
Standard level spoon measurements
are used in all recipes.
1 tablespoon = one 15 ml spoon
1 teaspoon = one 5 ml spoon

Both U.S. customary and metric
measurements have been given
in all recipes. Use one set of
measurements only and not a
mixture of both.

Eggs should be medium unless
otherwise stated.

Milk should be whole milk unless
otherwise stated.

Fresh herbs should be used unless
otherwise stated. If unavailable use
dried herbs as an alternative but
halve the quantities stated.

Ovens should be preheated to
the specified temperature – if
using a convection oven, follow
manufacturer's instructions for
adjusting the time and the
temperature.

Pepper should be freshly ground
black pepper unless otherwise stated.

Safety Note
It is advisable to check with your
doctor before embarking on any
exercise or diet program. *Home
Health Spa* should not be considered
a replacement for professional
medical treatment; a physician should
be consulted in all matters relating to
health and particularly in respect of
pregnancy and any symptoms which
may require diagnosis or medical
attention. While the advice and
information in this book is believed
to be accurate and the step-by-step
instructions have been devised to
avoid strain, neither the author nor
publisher can accept any legal
responsibility for any injury or illness
sustained while following the
exercises, treatments and diet plan.

contents

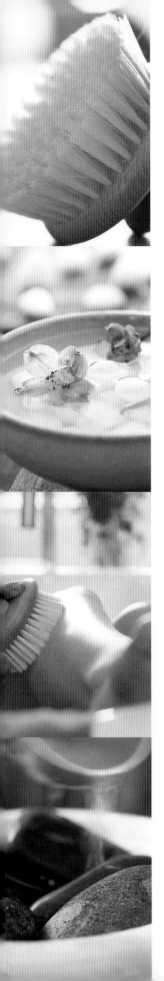

It is almost a cliché to say that most of us feel we are severely overstretched, trying to balance work, family commitments and a social life. All too often, the only thing most of us do not find time for is ourselves. Therefore, the idea of having a relaxing, pampered weekend is bound to appeal to everyone – just a couple of days where you come first. Many women, and quite a few men, are tempted by the thought of spending a weekend at a health spa. However, distance, time and, of course, money often make this out of the question. That is where *Home Health Spa* comes in. It shows you how to create your own spa at home, without spending a fortune.

The first thing you need to do is create an oasis of time. Choose a weekend that will be just for you, and don't make any other arrangements. Unplug the phone for the whole weekend and switch off the rest of the world. If you have children, ask your partner or a family member to take them for the weekend. Alternatively, you can always arrange a reciprocal weekend with other parents, who will have a free weekend when you take their children.

This does not mean you have to spend the whole time in isolation at home. Each of the three weekends includes at least one special treat, such as a visit to a professional therapist for a massage, or an afternoon at the local pool for a swim and a sauna. Apart from this, you should make sure you get out for a breath of fresh air every day. Take a walk, go cycling or do some gardening. You will find that the daily schedules will allow time for these activities.

You may also want to ask a friend to have a weekend spa with you. You can compare notes on how you are feeling as you progress.

However you decide to spend it, the most important thing is to relax and enjoy yourself, and not feel guilty about spending time on what you are doing. There will be very real benefits, even after this short period, and many of the techniques and therapies you make use of on each of the weekends may become part of your regular routine.

introduction

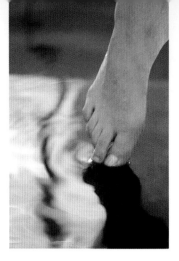

Home Health Spa is divided into three sections consisting of three programs, each with its own aims and benefits, and each occupying an entire weekend. Therefore, the first consideration is what you feel you need and what you want to achieve.

The Relaxing Weekend is for those who are experiencing prolonged stress. This can manifest itself in any number of ways – anxiety, headaches, digestive problems, depression, skin eruptions – or simply feeling unable to cope. By the end of this weekend, you should have brought both the physical and emotional symptoms of stress under control and be feeling rested and calm.

The Detoxing Weekend is deeply cleansing and restorative for body and mind. This is the weekend for you if you feel you have a poor diet of rich or junk foods or too much alcohol, or if you are continually battling against a polluted smoky atmosphere. It is also very helpful if you have decided to stop smoking; you will feel so purified by the end of the weekend, you may be very reluctant to spoil it all with a cigarette.

The Energizing Weekend is ideal when you feel under par. You may keep coming down with colds or flu, or feel tired all the time. This weekend boosts the immune system, makes you mentally alert and gives you extra energy.

Whichever program you decide to try, make sure you read through the whole program well in advance. Do all of your shopping the week before. You can also do some of the cooking in advance and put ready-prepared meals in the freezer to use as you need them. There may be other preparations, too. For example, you might want to make a relaxation tape for the relaxation weekend, or book a session with a massage therapist as your special treat. Most importantly, tell everyone you are unavailable that weekend. It is just for you.

Each weekend has a detailed schedule for you to follow. The chapter contents follow the schedule, but where elements are repeated over a weekend, you will need to refer back to an earlier page. Of course, these are your weekends, so feel free to adapt the schedule if you like.

how to use
this book

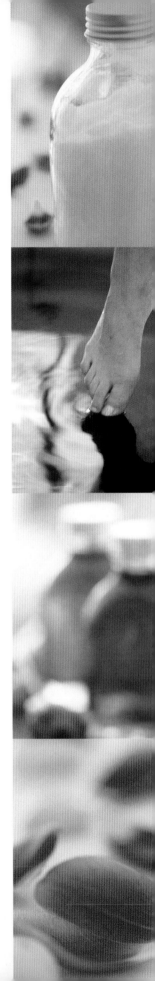

friday

7:00 pm
Evening meal

8:00 pm
Visualization

9:00 pm
Moor mud treatment

10:00 pm
Bed

5:00 pm
Herb tea or water

6:00 pm
Visualization

6:30 pm
Juice

8:00 pm
Herb tea or water

10:00 pm
Bed

saturday

8:00 am
Juice

9:00 am
Skin brushing and herb tea
or water

9:30 am
Hydrotherapy

10:30 am
Juice

11:00 am
Pilates

12:00 pm
Juice

2:00 pm
Herb tea or water

3:00 pm
Manual lymphatic drainage

4:00 pm
Juice

sunday

8:00 am
Body toning

9:00 am
Breakfast

11:00 am
Swim, sauna and steam

1:00 pm
Lunch

3:00 pm
Hair and skin cleanse

6:00 pm
Evening meal

8:00 pm
Epsom bath

10:00 pm
Bed

The Weekend

Because this weekend's cleansing diet depends on fresh,
preferably organic, fruit and vegetables, buy these on
Thursday or Friday so that they are at their best. Keep them in
the fridge until you need them. A skin brush and Moor mud
should be available from your local drugstore or health shop.
Don't forget to book your lymph massage session if you are
going to a professional and the sauna and steam rooms for
Sunday, if you need to do this in advance.

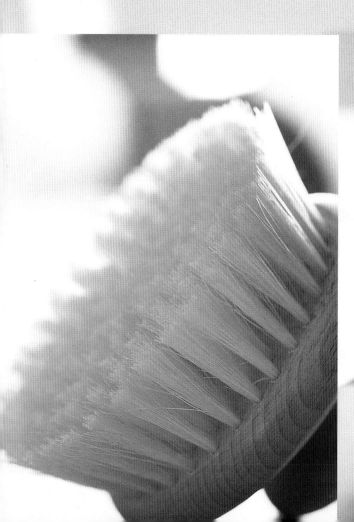

detoxing
weekend

friday

7:00 pm
Evening meal

8:00 pm
Visualization

9:00 pm
Moor mud treatment

10:00 pm
Bed

friday 7:00 pm **evening meal**

You begin your detox tonight. From now on, throughout the rest of the weekend, you will be eating and drinking only fresh and, if possible, organic fruit and vegetables. Because this is such a deeply cleansing diet, you will be throwing off toxins at quite a rate, so you may experience some unexpected side effects. These can include headaches, skin eruptions, a coated tongue, and strange smelling urine. You may also feel tired. None of these is anything to worry about. Take it easy as much as possible and, if you do get a headache, put some lavender oil in a burner and rest to ease it, rather than taking aspirin or analgesics.

After your supper, therapeutic bath and visualization session, go to bed early, allowing the body to get started on the detox without any distractions.

Salad supper

You begin the main detox tomorrow with a day of juice fasting. However, tonight you can eat.

Make yourself a big plate of salad, choosing from one of these recipes. Eat slowly, savoring the fresh flavors. Allow plenty of time for your food to digest by relaxing in a peaceful atmosphere. Part of the aim of this weekend is that your mind should free itself of all negative, stressful thoughts. To achieve this, you need to reverse the all too common feeling that we need to be going at full throttle all the time.

You should also start to increase your liquid intake tonight. Drink plenty of bottled or filtered water, or herb tea, throughout the evening. This will help to flush out the system and get the detoxing process off to a good start.

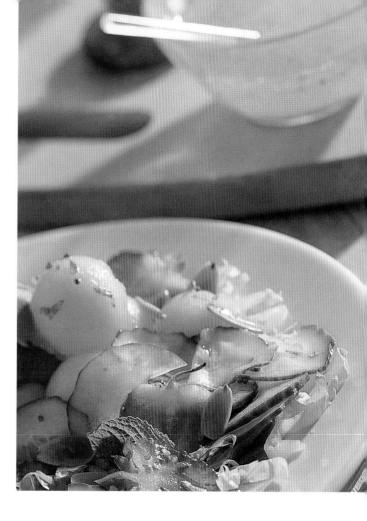

salads

Midsummer salad

Serves 1

¹/2 ripe cantaloupe
2 cups (0.275 liter) mixed
   baby greens, shredded
4–5 small strawberries, thinly
   sliced
1 inch (2.5 cm) piece of
   cucumber, thinly sliced
1 tablespoon chopped mint
1 tablespoon slivered
   almonds, to garnish
French dressing:
4 tablespoons olive oil
2 tablespoons white wine
   vinegar
¹/4 teaspoon French mustard
¹/2 garlic clove, chopped
1 teaspoon clear honey
small strip of lemon rind
few sprigs of herbs
salt
pepper

1 To make the dressing, beat together all the ingredients until well blended.

2 Cut the melon into quarters, remove the seeds and rind. Cut the flesh into cubes, or use a melon scoop to make balls.

3 Place the shredded lettuce on the plate, arrange the melon, strawberries and cucumber on top.

4 Mix the mint into the dressing and pour it over the salad. Serve garnished with almonds.

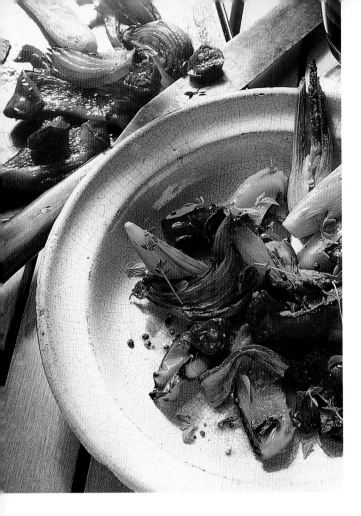

Mediterranean salad with grilled vegetables

Serves 1

1 small fennel bulb
1 red onion
2 zucchini, thinly sliced
   lengthways
2 tablespoons extra virgin
   olive oil
1/2 teaspoon finely grated
   lemon rind
1 teaspoon chopped thyme
1/2 red or yellow pepper,
   cored, deseeded and cut
   into strips
31/2 oz (100 g) cherry
   tomatoes, halved
Dressing:
2 tablespoons extra virgin
   olive oil
1 tablespoon lemon juice
pinch of sugar (optional)
1 teaspoon chopped
   oregano
salt
pepper

1 Cut the fennel bulb and
red onion into thick
wedges, leaving the root
ends intact to prevent them
falling apart while they
are cooking.

2 Bring a saucepan of water
to a boil. Add the fennel and
onion. When the water
returns to boiling, cook the
vegetables for 1 minute. Add
the zucchini strips and cook
for 1 minute more.

3 Drain in a colander and
refresh under cold running
water. Drain thoroughly and
set aside.

4 Combine the olive oil,
lemon rind and thyme in a
large bowl. Add the drained
vegetables, the pepper strips
and the cherry tomatoes.
Toss lightly to coat the
vegetables in the oil.

5 Line a broiler pan with
kitchen foil. Place the
vegetable mixture in it,
spreading evenly in a single
layer. Cook under a
preheated broiler for 15–20
minutes, turning frequently,
until the vegetables are
tender and patched with
brown. Allow the vegetables
to cool. Arrange on a plate.

6 To make the dressing,
beat together all the
ingredients until well
blended, pour over the
vegetables and serve.

Grilled asparagus salad

Serves 1

8 oz (250 g) asparagus
2 tablespoons olive oil
1 oz (25 g) arugula
1 oz (25 g) mixed baby
    greens
1 spring onion, finely
    chopped
2 radishes, thinly sliced
salt
pepper
Dressing:
2 tablespoons extra virgin
    olive oil
1 tablespoon lemon juice
pinch of sugar (optional)
1 teaspoon chopped oregano
To garnish:
roughly chopped herbs, such
    as tarragon, parsley,
    chervil or dill
thin strips of lemon rind

1 Trim the asparagus and use a potato peeler to peel about 2 inches (5 cm) off the base of each stalk.

2 Arrange the asparagus spears in a single layer on a baking sheet and brush them with olive oil. Cook under a preheated broiler for about 7 minutes, turning frequently, until the spears are just tender when pierced with the point of a sharp knife and lightly patched with brown.

3 Sprinkle the asparagus with salt and pepper and leave to cool.

4 Arrange the asparagus, arugula and mixed baby greens on a plate, with the spring onion and radishes.

5 Whisk all the dressing ingredients together in a bowl and pour it over the vegetables.

6 Garnish with the chopped herbs and lemon rind strips.

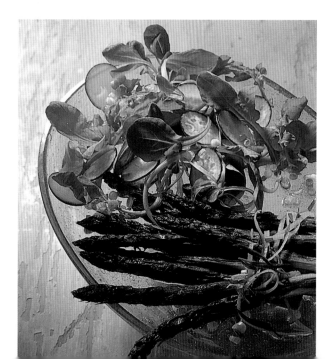

friday 8:00 pm **visualization**

Visualization is a form of meditation. Like all meditation, it helps to calm and focus the mind and has many additional benefits: it can improve memory and concentration, relieve stress and any addictive tendencies. If you find yourself craving particular foods or nicotine this weekend, you may well find that visualization will help.

There are several forms that visualization can take, three of which are described below. As its name suggests, visualization is all about seeing an image in your mind's eye. You can achieve this in three ways: by focusing, mental visualization and color visualization.

Focusing on an object is a good introduction to meditation, as you can remind yourself of what you are doing every time your eye wanders from the object. Mental visualization skips the real object and goes straight to the mental image. Color visualization appeals to many people, as they find a color much easier to concentrate on than a more complex image. You may want to try all three methods during the course of the weekend, but keep to one approach each session.

Preparing for visualization

Just as with meditating, when you are in a visualization session, you need to be free from distractions. So unplug the phone and, if there are other people about, ask them to be as quiet as possible and to keep out of the room. However, having someone else with whom to do the visualization exercise can often prove beneficial, adding to the focused atmosphere. Wear loose, comfortable clothing, make sure the room is warm but not stuffy, and sit in a position you can hold for up to 20 minutes. You can sit on the floor with your legs crossed or sit in a chair; the most important consideration is to be comfortable and not to have to move during the session.

Before you begin, take a few minutes to settle yourself both physically and mentally. Make sure you are sitting comfortably, and then focus on your mind. There will probably be plenty of thoughts whizzing around in your head, but just watch them, don't get caught up with them. Then place them on one side to deal with when you have finished.

Ideally, your visualization session should last for 20 minutes. If, however, you find this too difficult at first, begin with 10 minutes and try to extend the session a little each time. There will be two sessions a day for the rest of the weekend and the cumulative effect is most beneficial. By the fifth session on Sunday evening you should find your mind is becoming much clearer and calmer. When the session is finished, don't jump up immediately. Remain seated for a few minutes, breathing slowly, and try to retain the tranquillity for the rest of the evening.

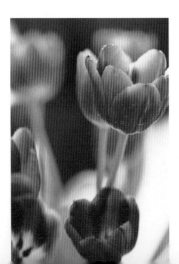

Focusing

Choose an object – something small and static, such as a flower, a stone or a lighted candle. Place this in front of you, preferably about 36 inches (90 cm) away and at eye level. Close your eyes and become aware of your body on the floor or chair. Become aware, too, of the noises around you – cars going by, dogs barking, babies crying. Simply observe these sounds and then let them go.

Open your eyes. Look, without blinking, at your chosen object for a minute, or as long as you can. Then close your eyes and look at the image it has left in your mind's eye. When the image fades, open your eyes and look again. Continue in this way, alternating real object with mental image, until the end of the session.

Mental visualization

Close your eyes and picture a place or an object, real or imagined, that you see solely with your mind's eye. Observe this in the greatest detail, focusing on it completely. A place of great tranquillity, such as a deserted beach, has a particularly calming influence.

Color visualization

Choose a color and, closing your eyes, try to fill your mind with it to the exclusion of everything else. It may be helpful to start by giving the color a picture – the blue sea, a snow scene or a field of golden corn. Then gradually try to go in closer so that you can no longer see the outlines of your picture and the color floods your mind.

friday 9:00 pm **moor mud treatment**

Mud may not be one of the most glamorous forms of treatment in the world, but it is certainly one of the oldest. Mud packs and masks were used by the ancient Egyptians and Romans for various ailments as well as beauty treatments, and were often given with other spa treatments as part of a cure. Therapeutic mud often comes from areas around mineral springs, and the high mineral content of the mud is regarded as one of the main reasons for its beneficial effects.

Mud treatments, like spas, are particularly popular in Europe. There, taking the waters (both drinking them and bathing in them) as well as all-over mud body wraps are frequently seen as important elements of a health regime and the annual spa "cure" is very much a part of everyday life. People may take cures for specific problems, such as arthritis or psoriasis, or as a more general detoxification.

Although mud treatments are now enjoying something of a revival, people have known of their therapeutic powers for a long period of time. One of the most famous sources of therapeutic mud is the Neydharting Moor, about 37 miles (60 km) from Salzburg in Austria. Archaeological finds on the moor have shown that it was in use from as early as 800 BC by the Celts and, later, the Romans. Sick and injured animals were, and still are, drawn there by its healing powers. Paracelsus, the 15th-century Swiss alchemist and physician, thought that he had discovered the elixir of life in mud. Later visitors included Louis XIV, Napoleon and Josephine, all of whom took the cure.

Known just as "Moor" or "Moor-Life," the mud has been investigated and analyzed by over 500 scientists, and has been found to be quite unique. Because the 20,000-year-old glacial valley basin in which it lies was first a lake and then a moor, the waters of which have never drained away, it has retained all of its organic, mineral and trace elements. Other moors have dried out and lost such substances, but clinical analysis has shown that the moor is uniquely rich in decomposed plant life, with over 1,000 plant deposits: flowering herbs, seeds, leaves, flowers, tubers, fruit, roots and grasses. Three hundred of them have recognized medicinal properties, and many of them are extinct or even unique to this one site.

Medical evidence shows Moor mud properties are both anti-inflammatory and astringent. This means it is particularly useful for detoxification, in treating skin disorders such as acne, eczema and psoriasis, and for rheumatism and arthritis. It is used, too, for beauty treatments, to remedy dry hair, and to reduce cellulite. Many health shops stock Moor mud treatments, and it is also available by mail order. (Search the Internet for suppliers.)

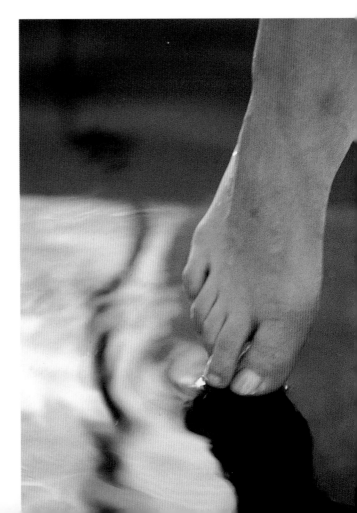

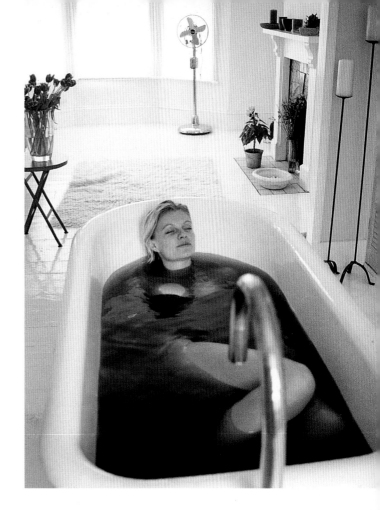

The Moor drink and Moor mud bath

The mud comes in a variety of forms, but the ones recommended here are the moor bath and the moor drink. Drinking mud does not sound very appetizing and, it has to be admitted, it does actually look like mud, which doesn't help. However, a teaspoonful mixed in a glass of water or fruit juice may color the liquid, but has neither taste nor odor. Take the drink about half an hour before you prepare for the Moor mud bath.

The best time for your bath is immediately before bedtime. Make sure the bathroom is warm, and run a deep bath, pouring in the Moor mud according to the instructions on the container. Mix it in well, or you will end up with muddy globules floating around in the water. Put some warm towels close to the bath to use when you come out.

Lie in the bath for 20–30 minutes. Splash the water on your face, too. You can also rinse it through your hair, if you don't mind having to dry it before you get into bed. Just try to relax in the bath, perhaps with some quiet music in the background. When you are ready to get out, pat yourself dry, but don't rub the towel over your skin. You want to leave as much residue from the bath on the surface of your skin as possible. Get into bed as soon as you are dry.

saturday

8:00 am	Juice
9:00 am	Skin brushing and herb tea or water
9:30 am	Hydrotherapy
10:30 am	Juice
11:00 am	Pilates
12:00 pm	Juice
2:00 pm	Herb tea or water
3:00 pm	Manual lymphatic drainage
4:00 pm	Juice
5:00 pm	Herb tea or water
6:00 pm	Visualization
6:30 pm	Juice
8:00 pm	Herb tea or water
10:00 pm	Bed

Today is the main day of your detoxing, with the juice fast at its center. Don't be too daunted by a liquid-only day; many people rather enjoy it. Fresh juice has a remarkably cleansing and regenerating effect on the entire system, as juices retain all of the nutrients that can be destroyed during the manufacturing process and during cooking. They are packed with anti-oxidants to accelerate healing and are low in calories. They are particularly effective at cleansing the gut. Juices are very easily assimilated by the body and contain all the nutrients present in raw fruit and vegetables, minus most of the fiber. Because it is easier to drink juice than it is to eat huge quantities of raw vegetables or fruit, you may find that you include a larger quantity of fresh, natural nutrients in your diet than usual.

You cannot make juice with a food processor or blender unless there is a separate juicing attachment. These machines will make a fruit or vegetable purée, while a juicer separates the fibrous pulp from the juice. If you do not have a juicer, you can purchase fresh juice in supermarkets or health food shops. Make sure they do not have any additives.

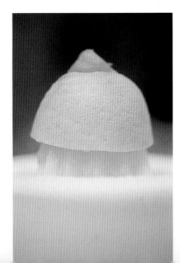

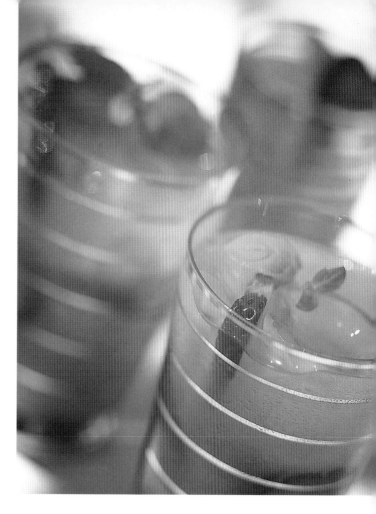

Preparing fruit and vegetables

Try to use organic fruit or vegetables and choose fruit that is ripe. It will be easier to juice and to digest. Don't buy bruised produce or produce that is obviously past its best. All fruit and vegetables, particularly non-organic, need to be very thoroughly cleaned, as you eat the entire thing. Leave on the tops and outer skins – many nutrients lie just below the surface of the skin. Remove peach stones but the smaller pips of apples can be juiced.

Homemade juice does not look the same as juice from a carton. It can have a rather murky-looking color, a much thicker consistency, sometimes with a froth on top, and a much more powerful taste. You don't need to strain the juice, even if it does have a froth. Give it a stir and drink it as soon as you have made it. Don't store any for later as it loses its nutritional value when it stands, even when kept in the fridge.

juices

If you have to purchase the juice, adapt the following menu according to availability. The recipes for the juices can be found on page 22.

- 8:00 am
  The juice of a lemon
  squeezed into hot water
- 9:00 am
  Herb tea or water
- 10:30 am
  Apple and carrot juice
- 12:00 pm
  Tomato juice
- 2:00 pm
  Herb tea or water
- 4:00 pm
  Raspberry and peach
  juice
- 5:00 pm
  Herb tea or water
- 6:30 pm
  Apple and carrot juice
- 8:00 pm
  Herb tea or water

Apple and carrot juice

Simply delicious, this juice is the best general tonic for cleansing and boosting the immune system. If you choose only one juice, this is the one.

4 carrots
2 green apples

Wash and chop the carrots and apples, if necessary, to fit in the juicer. Juice and drink immediately.

Raspberry and peach juice

Raspberry and peach juice is a thick, sweet, restorative juice. It is particularly good if you are overtired or anemic. If you find it too thick, add an apple or two.

8 oz (250 g) raspberries
2 peaches

Wash all the fruit and pit the peaches. Juice and drink immediately.

Tomato juice

This is a vivid, bright red juice. The tomatoes contain betacarotene, which helps to boost the body's immunity to disease.

6 tomatoes

Wash the tomatoes and cut them in half, if necessary, to fit in the juicer. Juice and drink immediately.

Topping up the liquids

Even though you are having nothing but liquid during the course of the day, juice alone will not be enough. You need to drink about 3 pints (1.8 liters) of extra fluids as well. Plenty of water, filtered or bottled, is most important. It helps to flush the toxins out of your system. If you want something warm, herb teas are an excellent way of increasing your fluid intake. They do not contain tannin or caffeine as they are made from pure herbs or, in some cases, spices. You can either make your own with herbs from the garden or supermarket or buy them ready-made. Whether you use fresh or dried herbs or tea bags, you should let them infuse for at least five minutes in boiling water before you drink them.

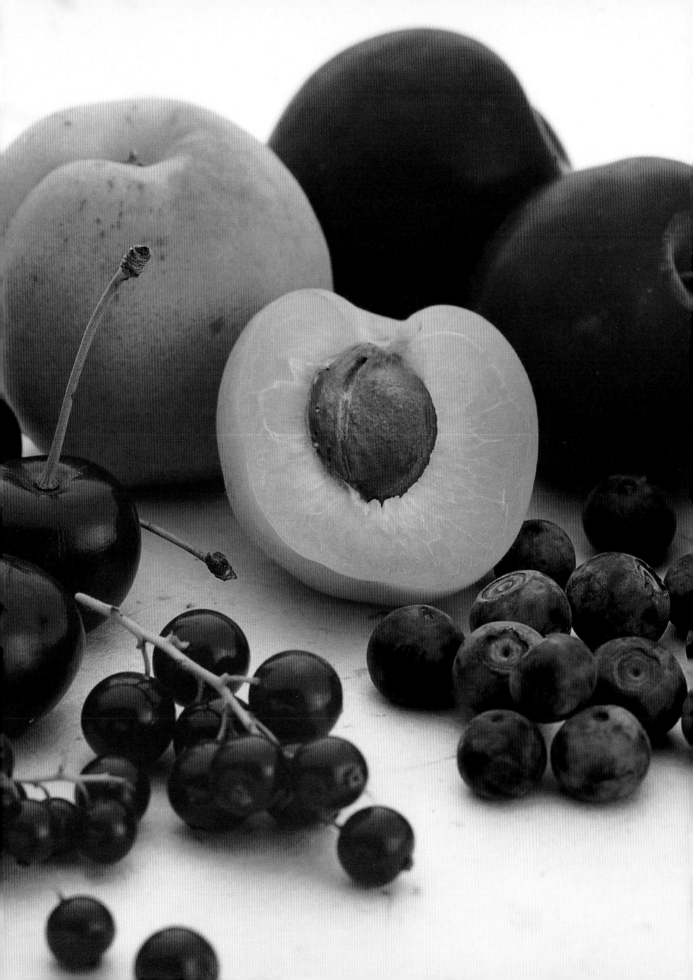

saturday 9:00 am **skin brushing**

The skin is the largest organ of the body, and the largest area from which toxins are eliminated. There are a number of treatments to stimulate this elimination, of which skin brushing is one. It improves the circulation of blood and lymph, which helps the body to slough off toxins more quickly and efficiently. Skin brushing makes the skin glow by removing the top dull, dead layer. The gentle massaging motion of the bristles also has a beneficial effect on areas of cellulite.

The technique is a simple one, and you need only a body brush with natural bristles or a loofah. There are various types of brushes, all widely available at drugstores. You will need a brush with a handle – some have detachable handles – so you can reach your back. There are also brushes mounted on long straps, which are ideal for the back and buttocks, and most loofahs are long enough to reach over the shoulders and down the back.

The method

Carry out skin brushing in the bathroom, as you will have your hydrotherapy shower and treatments immediately after. Skin brushing always comes first, as it is always done on dry skin. Make sure the bathroom is warm and there are plenty of towels. Undress, and find somewhere comfortable to sit so that you can easily reach your feet and lower legs.

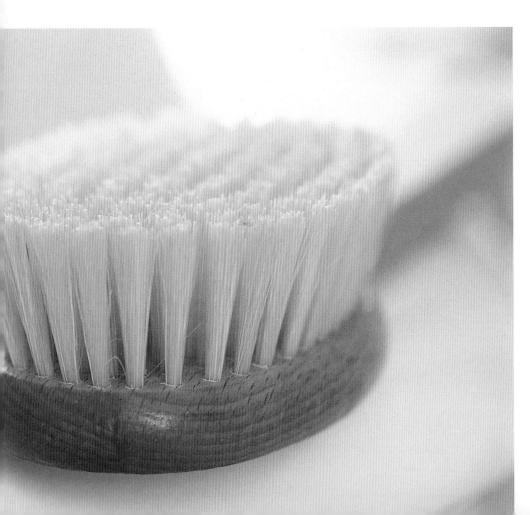

1 Take the brush and begin with the sole of your right foot. Use firm, rhythmic strokes to cover the sole several times. Next, brush the top of your foot, brushing up towards your ankle. Then go on to your lower leg, making sure you cover the whole surface – shin and calf. Always brush in an upward direction.

2 Stand up and brush the area from your knee to the top of your thigh. Make sure you cover the whole area several times, using long, rhythmic strokes. Brush your buttock area as far as your waist. Now repeat the whole procedure on your left leg, starting again with the sole of your foot.

3 Starting from the top of your buttocks, and always moving in an upward direction, brush the whole of your back several times all the way up to your shoulders.

4 Next, brush your right arm. Start with the palm of your hand, move on to the back of your hand and then brush from your wrist up to your elbow, always in an upward direction and ensuring that the whole surface of your skin is brushed. Brush your upper arm, always working from your elbow towards your shoulder, again covering the whole surface of your upper arm. Repeat on your left side, starting with your hand.

5 Very gently, brush your abdomen. Here, you brush in a circle, always in a clockwise direction. Cover the area several times but with less pressure than on your arms and legs. If it feels uncomfortable, stop.

6 The neck and chest are also very sensitive areas, so, again, brush here very gently. Always work towards your heart. If the bristles are too hard on your neck, don't brush here.

Brushing the whole body in this way will take between three and five minutes, depending on how many strokes you give to each area. Try to keep a rhythm going and brush for up to five minutes. If you do skin brushing on a daily basis, you will find a real improvement in your skin's texture – it tends to become very soft – and it will develop a rosy glow.

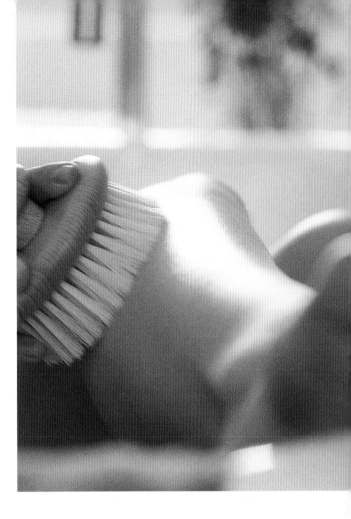

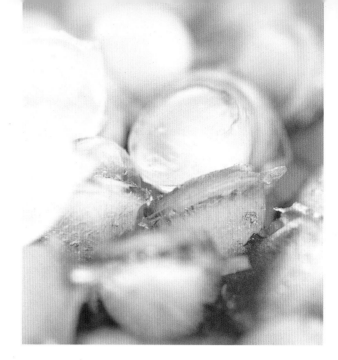

Hydrotherapy embraces a far-ranging collection of treatments using water. As with skin brushing, the effect of much hydrotherapy is to jump start the system, stimulating the circulation of the blood and lymph. This is often achieved by extremes of temperature, and you quite quickly become accustomed to it. Saunas, steam baths and Epsom baths are all aspects of hydrotherapy, but you begin the morning with a shower.

saturday 9:30 am hydrotherapy

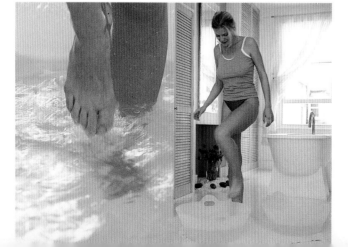

Hydrotherapy shower

The bathroom must be warm while you have this shower, and there should be plenty of warm towels at hand for when you finish. Begin by showering for two minutes in warm to hot water. Turn under the shower to make sure your whole body is covered in the water. Now turn the tap to cold and, again, turn your body under the shower so it covers you for 30 seconds. Turn the water back to hot for another two minutes, then to cold for a further 30 seconds. Repeat the whole process once more, finishing on cold. Turning your head so that the cold water pours on to your face is very beneficial for your complexion.

Get out and wrap yourself in warm towels. Pat yourself dry and put on a warm dressing gown. Sit or lie down for at least 10 minutes.

If you find the shower quite tiring, rest until it is time for body toning. However, if you find it stimulating, you might want to try one or two other hydrotherapy treatments. They are very beneficial during detoxification and will often give you a boost if you are feeling tired. If you wish, try one of the following.

Sitz bath

This treatment works on the same principle as the alternating of hot and cold water in the shower. Here, however, you are sitting in water. You need two bowls – washing-up bowls or bowls of a similar size.

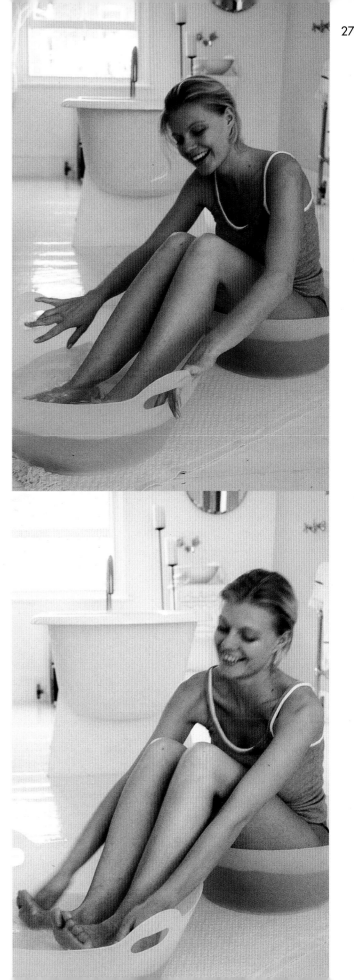

1 Fill one bowl with cold water; it should be very cold, so if you are feeling daring you could even put ice cubes in it. Fill the other with hot water (but test first, you do not want it so hot that you scald yourself).

2 You can wear a top during this treatment to keep your upper body warm, but it should not be so long that it falls into the water and gets wet. Start with your bottom in the hot water and then place your feet in the cold. This will be quite a shock to the system at first, but after a minute or two, you will start to feel quite comfortable. After five minutes, change over bowls so that your bottom is in the cold water and your feet are in the hot. Dry yourself, wrap up in a dressing gown or get into bed and rest.

Water treading

This involves somewhat less of a shock to the system than the last treatment as it only involves the feet. Wrap up to keep the body as warm as possible, but make sure your clothing does not extend beyond the knees. Your feet and lower legs should be bare.

Fill the bath with cold water, again making it as cold as possible. Now step into the bath and walk in the water on the spot, lifting your foot out of the water after each step. (Take care that the bath is not slippery. Put a rubber mat on the bottom if it is.) Tread water like this for one or two minutes. Get out of the bath, dry your feet well and put on warm socks. Rest afterwards for at least 10 minutes.

saturday 11:00 am **pilates**

When fasting, even for one day, over-energetic exercise is not appropriate, but a certain amount of gentle exercise will help the detoxification process and also make you feel good. People often assume that while they are fasting they will spend all of their time relaxing. In fact, if you were to lie in bed all day, your system would become sluggish, which is exactly the opposite of what you need while detoxing. Exercise also lifts the spirits, so it helps, too, to overcome feelings of tiredness or lethargy.

The exercises here are based on the Pilates technique, which is a very focused form of exercise. You concentrate on using specific muscle groups correctly to tone, strengthen and elongate and at the same time release tension and improve posture. Wear loose, comfortable, preferably cotton clothing for exercising, and use a room that is warm but not stuffy.

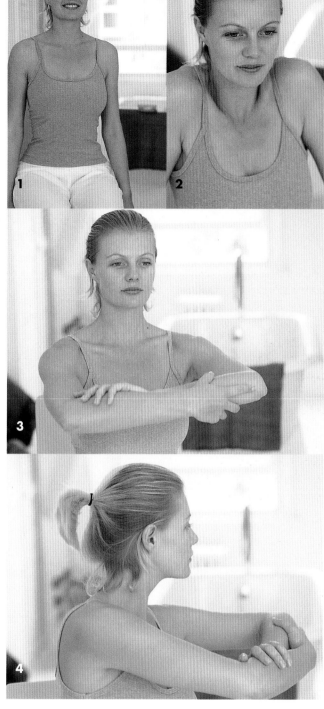

Opening up the upper body

1 Sit on a chair so that your knees are bent at right angles to your thighs when your feet are flat on the floor. Sit with a straight, long back and with your head held high. Focus straight ahead and let your arms hang by your sides. Pull in your stomach muscles and tense the muscles all around your ribs and waist.

2 Lift your shoulders up as high as you can, then let them drop right down – don't just place them down.

3 Fold your arms loosely in front of you at the height of your breastbone. Your hands should be relaxed, not gripping the arms. Breathe in and, as you breathe out, draw your navel gently towards your spine and start to turn from the waist.

4 Turn as far as you can to the side, leading with your elbows and making sure that the turn is from the waist only. Your hips stay absolutely still. Turn your head to follow the movement. When you have turned as far as you can, breathe in and return to the center. Repeat on the other side, then alternate until you have turned each way 10 times.

Strengthening the abdominals

1 Lie on your back with your knees raised, feet flat on the floor. Your entire spine should be flat on the floor as well. Make sure it is completely straight and that your neck is long, with no tension in your shoulders. Let your arms lie comfortably at your sides.

2 Take a deep breath and, as you breathe out, draw your navel to your spine so that you become aware of the small of your back on the floor. Squeeze the muscles at the base of your buttocks, not your thighs. Then very slowly start to curl up off the floor, bringing your buttocks and your lower back up in a scooped-out shape. You should have no tension in the shoulders or neck, which stay relaxed on the floor throughout. Only come up as far as you can. If your abdominal muscles quiver or bulge out, you have come too far. Keeping the movement very slow and focused, repeat up to 10 times.

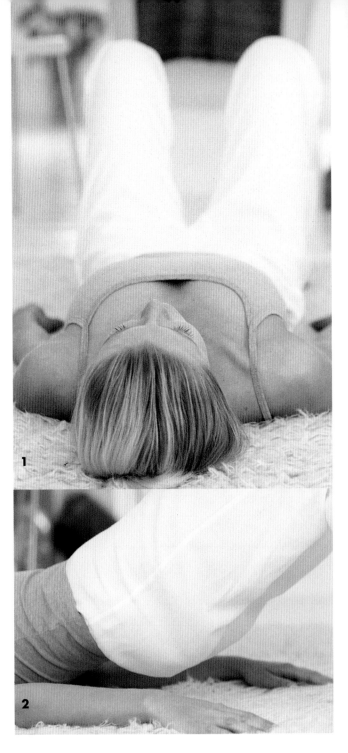

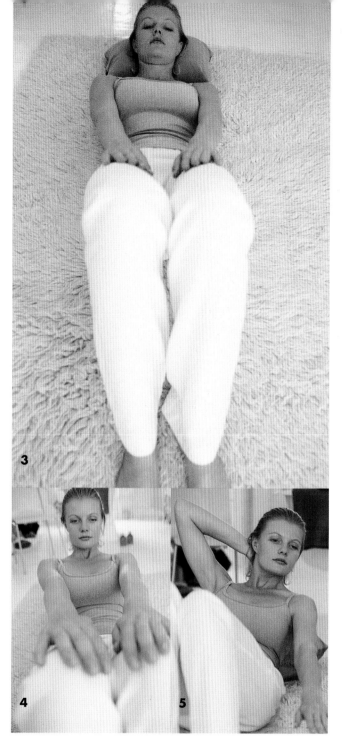

3 Lie on the floor in the same position as step 1. Put a cushion under your head and shoulders if this feels more comfortable. Place your hands on your thighs.

4 Breathe in and, as you breathe out, press your navel to your spine and slowly start to slide your fingers up your thighs towards your knees. As you do so, your head and shoulders will start to curl up off the floor. Don't expect to come up too high. It is more important to use the muscles correctly than to come up a long way off the floor. Again, if your abdominal muscles bulge or quiver, you have come too high.

● When your fingers have reached as far as they can, place your hands flat on your thighs again, breathe in, and slide your hands down, uncurling back down on to the floor. Repeat this exercise up to 10 times.

5 Lie in the same starting position as step 4 and, this time, place your right hand under your head and your left arm on the floor at your side.

● Breathe in and, as you breathe out, press your navel to your spine and slowly reach your left hand down the floor towards your feet. This will make your head and left shoulder curl off the floor. Only go as far as you can, maintaining the concave navel. Curl back down to the floor and repeat, reaching to the right. Build up to 10 repetitions on each side.

Toning the legs and buttocks

1 Lie on your right side with your back flat against a wall. Stretch your right arm above your head and place your head on it, with a cushion if you feel more comfortable. Make sure your left leg makes one long line with your body. Bend your right knee in front of you.

2 Breathe in and, as you breathe out, stretch your left leg away from you in a long, low lift, keeping the whole of your back flat against the wall. Check with your left hand that your hip doesn't move. Breathe in and lower. Repeat slowly 10 times, then repeat on the right leg.

3 Now bend your top leg, keeping your back flat against a wall. Straighten the lower leg so that it is in line with the body.
● Breathe in and, as you breathe out, press your navel to your spine and lift the lower leg slowly up and down. Now repeat with the other leg. Work up to 10 repetitions on each side.

Arm toners

1 Lie on your back, knees lifted and feet flat on the floor, slightly apart. The whole spine should be long and touching the floor, with no tension in the neck or shoulders. Hold a weight of around 2 lb (1 kg) in each hand and place your arms out to the side.

2 Lift your arms up so that they form a wide circle, as if they were reaching around a huge ball. Breathe in and, as you breathe out, draw your navel down towards your spine. Breathe in and open your arms out to the side, still keeping the curved shape. Breathe out and return, repeating 10 times.

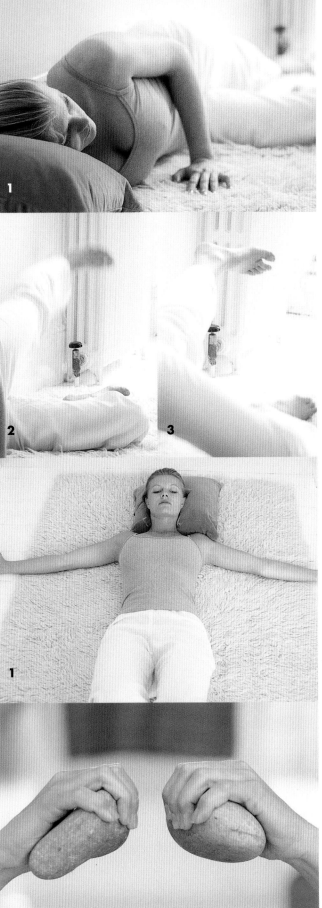

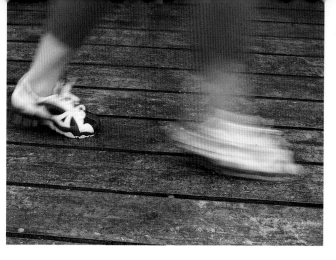

saturday 3:00 pm **manual lymphatic drainage**

Any type of massage will help you to relax. However, for this weekend, one in particular is of the greatest help in the actual process of detoxification, as well as contributing to a feeling of well being. Known as Manual Lymphatic Drainage (MLD), this is a very gentle, rhythmical technique which, by stimulating the lymphatic system, accelerates the process of shedding toxins. MLD is now widely available. If your local health club, gym or pool offers massage, ask if any of the therapists have trained in MLD and book an appointment to give yourself a treat.

The lymphatic system resembles the circulation system, with the major difference that it does not have a central organ, like the heart in the circulatory system, to keep the lymph moving. Rather, the lymph moves as a result of the muscles contracting and relaxing, hence the beneficial effects of exercise on the lymphatic system. Keeping the lymph moving is vital because it plays such a central part in the health of the immune system. Essentially, it is the body's waste disposal system. It gets rid of toxins and dead cells, particles of pollution and antibiotics. So, by stimulating the lymphatic system, detoxification becomes more efficient, too.

Manual lymph drainage, by accelerating the workings of the lymphatic system, reduces many of the symptoms that are caused when it is overstretched. These include bloating,

cellulite and premenstrual tension. It is also an extremely relaxing therapy, and the very gentle strokes that are used make it ideal during fasting when you may be feeling particularly sensitive.

If you are unable to find an MLD therapist, there are some very effective ways of stimulating the lymphatic system. One is rebounding – jumping on a mini-trampoline – for about 10–15 minutes. Alternatively, a brisk walk is an excellent way of stimulating the lymph. The more pleasant the surroundings, the better the walk. Go to the country, a lake or a park. Wear loose, comfortable clothes and low-heeled shoes. Walk at a brisk pace, but don't try jogging. Enjoy your surroundings, breathe deeply and spend at least an hour walking.

Following this, spend the rest of the day relaxing. Between resting and juices, you should fit in another visualization session for 20 minutes. Before bed, you can, if you wish, have a relaxing bath to put you in the mood for a restful night's sleep. Try either the Moor mud bath from Friday night (see pages 18–19) or the Epsom bath (see page 47). Alternatively, if you would like something a little more sensual, you could try the aromatherapy bath from the Relaxing Weekend (see pages 56–57). Whatever you decide, aim to be in bed by about 10 pm.

sunday

8:00 am	Body toning
9:00 am	Breakfast
11:00 am	Swim, sauna and steam
1:00 pm	Lunch
3:00 pm	Hair and skin cleanse
6:00 pm	Evening meal
8:00 pm	Epsom bath
10:00 pm	Bed

Today you will be eating solid food, but the detoxification will continue as you are eating only raw food, and some very lightly cooked fruit and vegetables. Drink just as much water as yesterday and include herbal teas whenever you like. The greater the quantity of these fluids you drink, the quicker the toxins will be flushed through the system.

Any fruit is good for breakfast. You can just mix up whatever appeals to you and looks good when you go shopping. Try to buy organic produce whenever possible and make sure it is ripe and therefore at its most delicious. You can have fruit juice and a herb tea to drink. The following are a few alternatives.

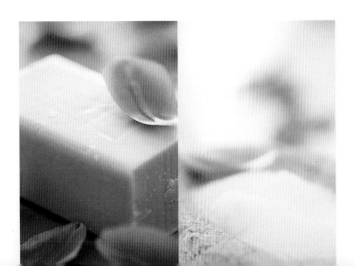

Tropical temptation

1 mango
1/2 pineapple, or 1 small
   pineapple
6 strawberries
4 tablespoons pineapple
   juice
honey, to taste (optional)

1 Peel the mango and the pineapple and cut them into cubes, discarding the pineapple core. Hull the strawberries.

2 Pour the pineapple juice over the fruit and leave to soak for 30 minutes. If the fruit is ripe this should sweeten it enough. However, if it is too tart for your taste, add a little honey.

Stuffed figs

3 ripe figs
1 tablespoon ground
   almonds
1 oz (25 g) raspberries
honey, to taste (optional)

1 Remove the stalks from the figs, make a criss-cross cut at the stalk end and carefully ease them open.

2 Mix the almonds and raspberries together and spoon them into the open figs, adding a little honey to sweeten if you wish.

Kiwi fruit and ginger cup

1/2 cantaloupe, deseeded
1 kiwi fruit, thinly sliced
8 oz (250 g) green grapes,
   halved
1/2 teaspoon grated
   gingerroot
4 tablespoons apple juice

1 Cut the melon piece in half, remove the seeds and rind. Cut the flesh into cubes, or use a melon scoop to make balls.

2 Place the melon, kiwi fruit and grapes in a bowl. Scatter with the ginger and then pour the juice over the fruit. Serve immediately.

breakfasts

sunday 11:00 am
swim, sauna and steam

Sunday's hydrotherapy takes you out to your local gym or swimming pool. Ideally, you should look for a leisure center or health club that has a swimming pool, sauna and steam room. You can, however, improvise. The other alternative, if you don't have a local pool, or you simply don't feel like going out, is to repeat yesterday's hydrotherapy at home.

Swimming

Swimming is the ideal exercise for a detoxing weekend. You use most of the muscle groups in your body if you vary your strokes, but your muscles and joints are supported by the water, so you are not going to injure yourself, as you might do in an overly energetic aerobics class. It is not necessary to swim at a furious pace or for a long period of time and, if you alternate swimming with the other hydrotherapy methods, your mind and body will feel completely relaxed afterwards.

You can also do some exercises in the water that are particularly beneficial if your joints are stiff. They also help to improve muscle tone, as you are working against the resistance of the water. Warm up first with a couple of lengths and, if you start to feel cold, have another swim.

Exercises for legs and hips

1 Stand so that your side is next to the edge of the pool and hold on to the handrail. With a straight back, lift your outside leg and swing it back and forth as far as you can. Do this 10 times, then change legs.

2 Walk on the spot, feeling your feet go down through your toes to your heels every time you replace them on the floor of the pool. Gradually make the steps bigger, with your knees coming higher each time. If you can, after two minutes, turn this into a run. Continue running for two minutes.

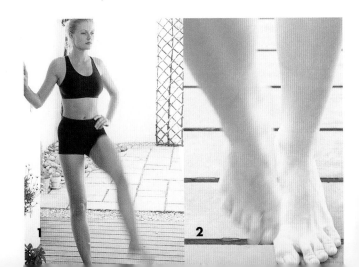

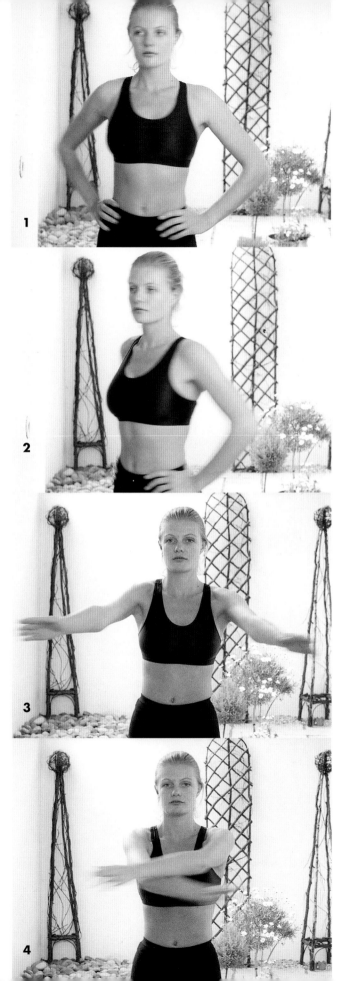

Exercises for the upper body

1 Standing away from the edge of the pool, with your feet apart, put your hands on your hips.

2 Turn as far as you can to the right and then to the left. Repeat 10 times, alternating from side to side.

3 With your shoulders under the water (you can kneel for this if the water is very shallow) take your arms out to your sides so that they are just under the water.

4 With a slight curve from shoulder to your wrist, slowly bring your hands together against the resistance of the water. When your forearms meet, there should be a large circle of water between your arms – enough to encompass a beach ball. Slowly repeat the exercise 10 times.

Sauna and steam

Alternating saunas and steam baths with a cold shower or a swim in the pool works on the hydrotherapy principle of stimulating the circulation of blood and lymph by changing the temperature. Of course, you sweat off waste in the sauna or steam bath, too, which helps the detoxification process further.

Many health clubs have saunas and steam baths. If you have a pool with a sauna or a steam bath adjacent, this is ideal. However, do remember that a very light diet combined with sudden changes of temperature may make you a little light-headed, so move from one to the other slowly. If you want to have a fairly lengthy swim, do this first.

If for some reason you can only do this in the afternoon, make sure at least two hours have passed since your last meal. Take off all your jewelry and, for maximum benefit, wear as little as possible.

Alternate five to ten minutes of heat with one or two lengths of the pool, and repeat this a few times. If you don't have a pool, have a cool to cold shower and rest for a few minutes before returning to the heat treatment. Drink plenty of water throughout. Dry yourself gently, then rest, lying down, before you get dressed and go home.

salads

Lunch and evening meal

Sunday's lunch and evening meal are salads. If you can, eat at least one salad meal a day for the week following your detox and drink plenty of water; this will allow the cleansing process to continue. All of the recipes here are for four small or two large servings. You can, of course, have two smaller salads at the same meal.

Continental mixed salad

1 red oakleaf lettuce, separated into leaves
1/2 head of frisé lettuce (chicory), separated into leaves
2 oz (50 g) arugula
2 oz (50 g) mixed baby greens
handful of herbs, such as dill, chives and basil
1 red onion, thinly sliced
1 large, ripe avocado
1 tablespoon lemon juice
1 oz (25 g) pine nuts, toasted
handful nasturtium flowers (optional)
salt
pepper
1 recipe of tarragon dressing (see potato and celery salad, opposite)

1 Tear the oakleaf leaves and the frisé into bite-size pieces. Put them in a large salad bowl with the arugula, mixed baby greens, herbs and red onion.

2 Peel, halve and stone the avocado. Roughly chop the flesh and place in a small bowl with the lemon juice. Toss gently.

3 Just before serving, add the avocado, pine nuts and flowers to the salad and season with salt and pepper to taste. Spoon the tarragon dressing over the salad and toss gently.

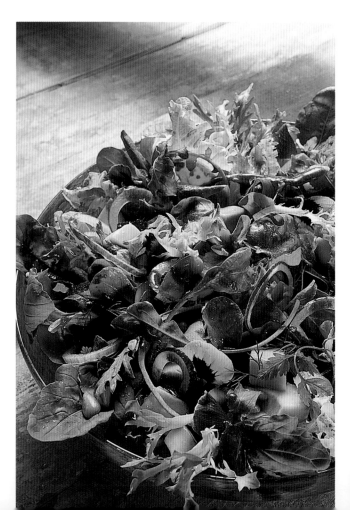

Potato and celery salad

1 lb (500 g) small white or
    yellow potatoes, scrubbed
6 celery sticks, with leaves
3 oz (75 g) black olives
3 tablespoons capers, rinsed
    and drained
few sprigs of parsley, roughly
    chopped
salt
pepper
Tarragon dressing:
2 tablespoons tarragon
    vinegar
1 teaspoon finely grated
    lemon rind
1/4 teaspoon Dijon mustard
5 tablespoons olive oil
salt
pepper

1 Bring a saucepan of
water to a boil. Add the
potatoes and boil for about
12 minutes until just tender.
Drain and leave to cool.

2 Slice the celery sticks
diagonally and roughly
chop any leaves. Place in
a bowl with the olives,
capers and parsley. Add
the cooked potatoes and
season with salt and pepper
to taste.

3 To make the dressing,
beat together all the
ingredients until well
blended. Pour the dressing
over the salad, toss well
and serve.

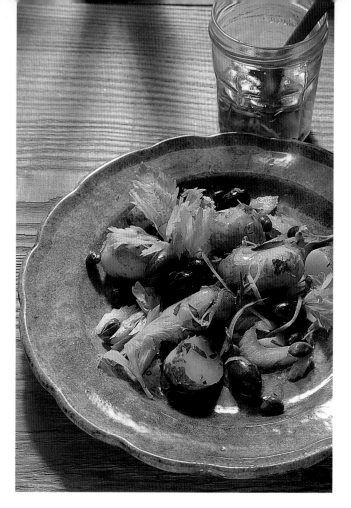

Mixed baby greens lettuce with mango and mint

1 large mango
1 tablespoon chopped mint
1 tablespoon lime juice
8 oz (250 g) mixed baby
    greens
4 oz (125 g) roasted
    cashew nuts
handful of nasturtium leaves
    and flowers, to garnish
    (optional)
Yogurt dressing:
1/4 pint (150 ml) natural
    yogurt
1 tablespoon lemon juice
1 teaspoon clear honey
1/2 teaspoon Dijon mustard
salt
pepper

1 Peel and stone the mango
and chop it into bite-size
pieces. Place them in a bowl
with the mint and lime juice
and mix well.

2 Place the mixed baby
greens in a salad bowl. Add
the prepared mango and the
cashew nuts.

3 To make the dressing, beat
together all the ingredients
until well blended. Drizzle the
dressing over the salad and
toss lightly. Garnish with
nasturtium leaves and flowers.

Cottage garden salad with strawberries

8 oz (250 g) mixed salad
   leaves, such as
   dandelion, arugula, red
   oakleaf, radicchio and
   mixed baby greens
handful of herbs, such as
   fennel, chives, dill and
   mint
8 oz (250 g) small
   strawberries
1 recipe tarragon dressing
   (see potato and celery
   salad, page 39)
salt
pepper

1 Tear the lettuce leaves into
pieces and place them in a
salad bowl. Scatter the herbs
over the lettuce.

2 Halve the strawberries and
add them to the salad with a
little salt and pepper.

3 Spoon the dressing over
the salad and toss lightly.

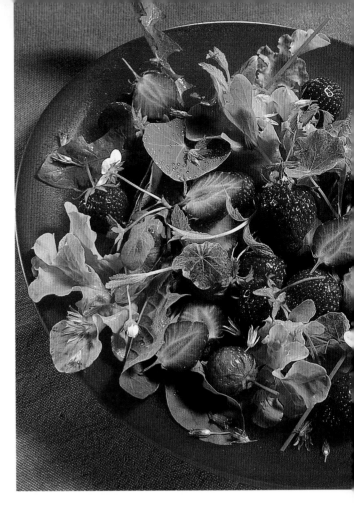

salads

French bean and apricot salad

1 lb (500 g) French beans, trimmed
6 ripe apricots, halved, pitted and sliced
few sprigs of parsley, roughly torn
1 tablespoon chopped tarragon
1 recipe tarragon dressing (see potato and celery salad, page 39)
salt
pepper
1 oz (25 g) sliced almonds, toasted, to garnish

1 Cook the French beans for 2–3 minutes in a saucepan of boiling water. Drain well and place in a salad bowl.

2 Add the sliced apricots to the beans, then add the parsley and tarragon. Season with salt and pepper.

3 Pour the dressing over the salad and toss lightly. Garnish the salad with the sliced almonds and serve.

Green salad with walnuts

large bowl of mixed salad leaves, such as arugula, chicory and spinach
½ mild onion, chopped
2 oz (50 g) walnut pieces
Dressing:
1 recipe tarragon dressing (see potato and celery salad, page 39), substituting walnut oil for the olive oil

1 Tear the salad leaves roughly and put them in a serving bowl with the onion.

2 Lightly toast the walnuts in a dry pan. Chop them and leave to cool.

3 To make the dressing, beat together all the ingredients until well blended.

4 Add the walnuts to the salad and pour the dressing over the top. Toss lightly to mix.

Grilled pepper salad

2 red peppers
2 yellow peppers
2 green peppers
2 garlic cloves, chopped
1 tablespoon chopped parsley
2 sprigs of basil, shredded
5 tablespoons extra virgin olive oil
2 teaspoons balsamic vinegar
salt
pepper
basil leaves, to garnish

1 Preheat the broiler. Place the whole peppers on the broiler pan and cook, turning occasionally, until the skins are blistered and blackened all over. This will take about 20 minutes. Place the peppers in a paper or plastic bag and secure the top. Leave to cool.

2 When cool enough to handle, hold the peppers over a bowl to catch the juices and remove and discard the charred, papery skins. Remove and discard the core and seeds.

3 Cut the pepper flesh into long thin strips and arrange them in a shallow serving dish. Sprinkle the chopped garlic, parsley and basil over the peppers. Season with salt and pepper.

4 Drizzle the oil and balsamic vinegar over the salad and serve, garnished with basil leaves.

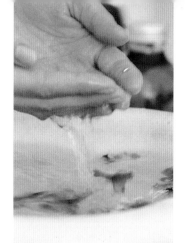

sunday 3:00 pm **hair and skin cleanse**

The afternoon treatment is a relaxing, deep cleanse for the hair and skin. It helps eliminate toxins, many of which are lost through the skin during detoxification. Keep drinking as much water as you can to speed up the process of flushing the toxins out of your body.

The hair treatment

Apply the hair treatment before you cleanse your face. It contains oily substances, so you will probably want to wash your hair once you have finished. Alternatively, leave it on all night and wash it off when you shower tomorrow morning. Choose the treatment according to your hair type, massage it in well, then wrap a towel around your head for the rest of the session. The treatment oils for greasy or dry and damaged hair appear on page 88.

A hair growth stimulant can be a beneficial treatment if your hair seems very thin or if you have lost hair because of childbirth, stress or as a reaction to illness or drugs. Put 10 drops of rosemary oil, 10 drops of lavender oil and 5 drops of sandalwood oil in 2 oz (50 ml) of carrier oil and massage it into your scalp.

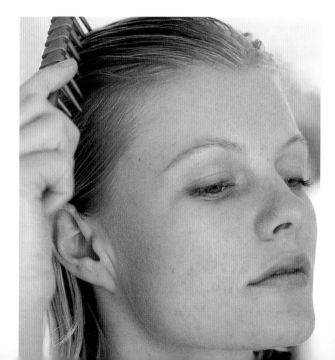

The facial cleanse

You can choose homemade or over-the-counter products for this deep cleansing facial, or a mixture of the two. Follow each stage carefully according to your skin type.

1 Cleanse your face and neck thoroughly to remove all traces of make-up and dirt and pollution from the atmosphere. Either use a cleanser that is applied with water or a cleansing lotion applied with cotton pads or balls. Do not use soap. If you use a cleanser that is applied with water, take a face buff (an object that is like a loofah for the face) and go all over your face using small circular movements to give your skin a mini-exfoliation.

2 Whichever cleansing method you have used, splash some cold water on to your face and neck about 20 times. Pat dry.

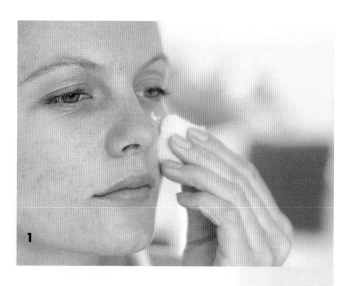

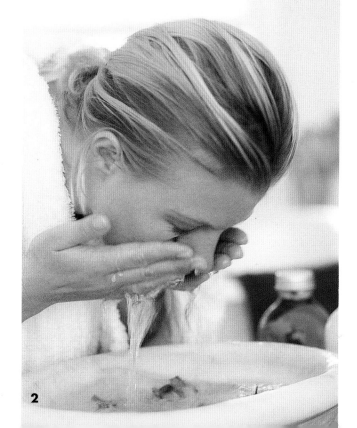

3 Exfoliating requires a grainy cleanser that penetrates deeper into the skin by removing all the dry, dead cells on the surface. There is a wide range of proprietary brand exfoliators, available as gels, liquids, creams and pastes. Choose one that goes on easily so that you don't end up dragging the skin. Alternatively, make your own by mixing together a teaspoonful each of live yogurt, crushed rolled oats and honey. Use small circular movements to cover your whole face and neck, and rinse off with warm water, splashing 20 times. Pat dry.

● Apply a cleansing mask to your face and neck, but not to your eye area. This will cleanse your face further, drawing out impurities, and close the pores. There are a vast number of over-the-counter masks available and you can choose one according to your skin type. If you prefer, make your own from natural ingredients (see page 88).

4 Apply a chamomile eye compress (see page 89) and lie down and relax.

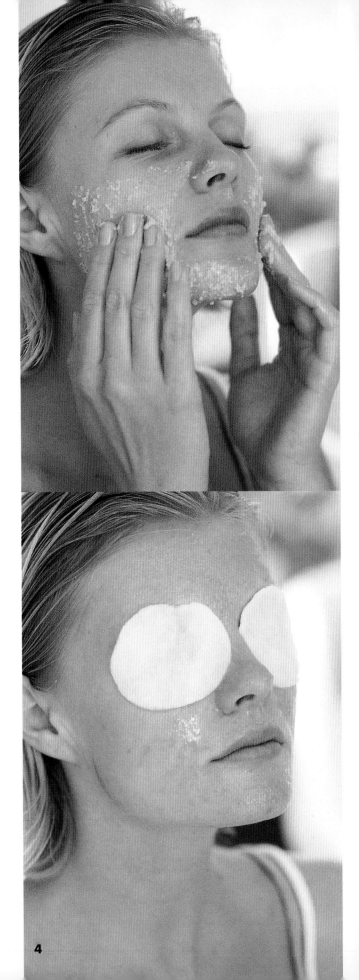

4

5 Rinse off the mask completely and spray with the gentle facial toner (see page 88). Apply a moisturizer (again, you can make your own aromatherapy version, try the essential oil skin conditioners on page 88) or simply spread a thin layer of petroleum jelly over your entire face and neck.

6 Relax until supper time.

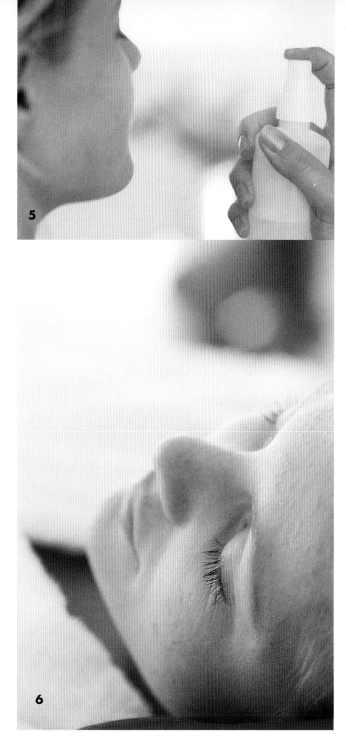

sunday 3:00 pm **hair and skin cleanse**

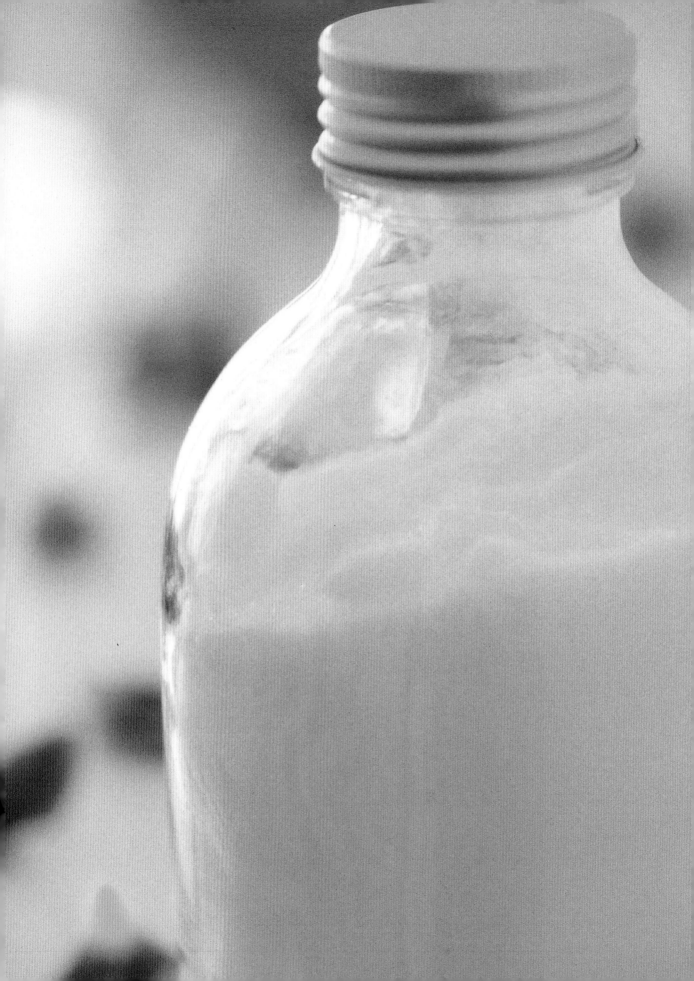

An Epsom salts bath probably does not sound like a very glamorous end to your weekend. However, it is one of the most cleansing and relaxing late-night treatments imaginable. This is because the magnesium in Epsom salts warms and soothes the body, so the joints and muscles relax. At the same time, you can expect to get very hot indeed – your temperature will rise and you will release extra toxins in the form of sweat.

Epsom salts are available at some drugstores and health food shops. If you have difficulty finding them, you can substitute herbs and spices; ginger, sage and cayenne pepper have a similar effect in terms of raising the body's temperature.

Caution: Do not use Epsom salts if you have eczema, psoriasis or broken skin. Take a soothing aromatherapy bath instead (see page 56).

The bathroom should be warm and you should have plenty of towels handy. The salts usually come in 4 lb (2 kg) packs, and you put the whole contents of the pack into the bath. It takes quite a lot of stirring to mix the salts into the water, but do make sure the entire contents of the container have dissolved before you get in.

Soak yourself in the bath for at least five minutes. You will start to sweat copiously. However, don't worry, this is completely normal and is part of the process that detoxifies and relaxes your body.

Use a loofah or bath mitt and, beginning with your feet, thoroughly massage with circular movements. Don't try to go too fast or you may become overheated. Work your way up your legs, massaging as you go, then kneel to work on your buttocks and your abdomen (go gently on the latter). Sit down and work gently over the lower half of your chest, avoiding your breasts, and working over as much as you can of your back.

Lie back and relax for another five minutes, if you can. If you find you are becoming too hot, step out of the bath immediately. Wrap yourself in towels and pat your body dry very gently. Do not rub your skin. When you are dry, get into bed and prepare for a long, restful night.

sunday 8:00 pm **epsom bath**

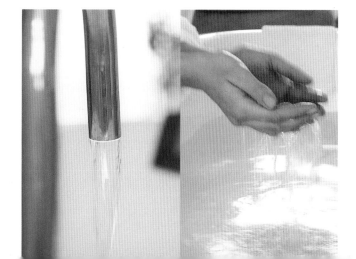

A certain amount of short-term stress is not such a bad thing; as a challenge, it can actually motivate us. However, in the long term it can cause all manner of physical and emotional ailments, from migraine and depression to eczema and irritable bowel syndrome.

One of the side effects of stress, and also one of its causes, is lack of time for yourself. You are so busy coping, you forget, or are unable, to relax. The point of this weekend is to reverse this trend. Not only will you give yourself time and several pampering treats, but you will also learn a number of techniques that help to combat stress. Ideally, these should be incorporated into your everyday life.

The Weekend

Look through the recipes for the weekend (see pages 52–55, 66–67 and 72–75) and make a list of the food and drink you need to buy in advance. It is a good idea to prepare as much as you can beforehand so you have as few chores as possible during the weekend itself. All of the soups, for example, can be made in advance and frozen until you are ready to use them. You can make your own relaxation tape the week before as well (see pages 68–71). If you decide to go out for a professional massage on Saturday, make sure you book your appointment well in advance.

friday

7:00 pm
Meditation

8:00 pm
Evening meal

9:00 pm
Aromatherapy bath

10:00 pm
Self-massage for sleep

saturday

8:00 am
Yoga

9:00 am
Breakfast

10:00 am
Relaxation and meditation

12:00 pm
Lunch

2:00 pm
Massage

4:00 pm
Facial massage

6:00 pm
Evening meal

8:00 pm
Breathing techniques and meditation

10:00 pm
Bed

sunday

8:00 am
Yoga, relaxation and meditation

9:00 am
Breakfast

11:00 am
Acupressure

1:00 pm
Lunch

3:00 pm
Aromatherapy facial

4:00 pm
Meditation

6:00 pm
Evening meal

8:00 pm
Aromatherapy bath

10:00 pm
Bed

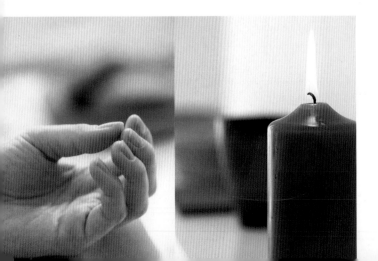

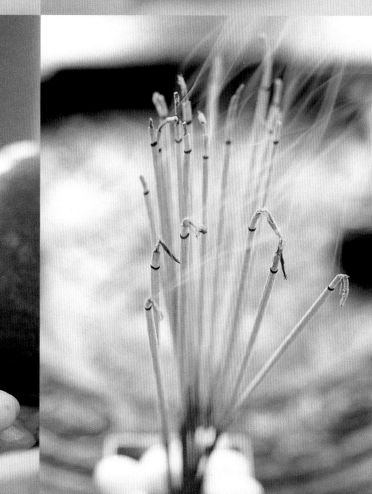

relaxing
weekend

friday

friday 7:00 pm **meditation**

There are numerous relaxation techniques that can overcome the immediate stresses and strains of contemporary life. However, a period of prolonged stress is another matter, manifesting itself as high blood pressure, raised cholesterol levels, anxiety, depression and insomnia. To overcome these problems, a quite different form of deep relaxation is needed to disperse severe stress of body and mind.

Regular meditation has emerged as the most effective way of achieving deep relaxation. A considerable body of clinical research, focusing mainly on the most dramatic and measurable manifestations of stress, such as heart disease, has shown that meditation results in substantial reductions in blood pressure and cholesterol levels. Other clinical tests have shown that the risk of much of the physical and mental deterioration associated with aging is reduced considerably by regular meditation. Meditation is not, however, merely a prophylaxis. Some of its other benefits include:

- physical relaxation
- improved concentration
- increased tranquillity and ability to deal with stress
- improved awareness
- improved creativity and memory

Preparing for meditation

Meditation is not just day-dreaming or relaxation. Primarily, it is a discipline for training your mind to a point of both deep concentration and relaxation. During this weekend, you can only hope to achieve an idea of what meditation is like. The first session may seem a little strange, but if you get into a regular rhythm of meditation during the course of these three days, you may well find that its benefits make it something you want to continue.

The main thing to remember when learning to meditate is that the intrusion of thoughts is inevitable. Do not try too hard; you are not supposed to be forcing your mind to concentrate on a particular image. In fact, you are trying to release yourself from conscious thought. When any thought enters your mind, observe its presence gently, make no judgement about the thought itself and, above all, do not become irritated with yourself for having it. Recognize the thought, let it go and draw your focus back to your breath or the word or image on which you are meditating.

You need to be comfortable but alert to meditate. You should also avoid being disturbed. Take the phone off the hook, find a quiet spot, wear loose, comfortable clothing and take off your shoes. You can sit in a straight-backed chair or cross-legged on the floor. The important thing is to sit with a straight back and remain still for up to 20 minutes.

Before you begin, take some slow, deep breaths and try to let go of any areas of tension. Scan your mind for immediate thoughts and worries, then leave them on one side so your mind is clear.

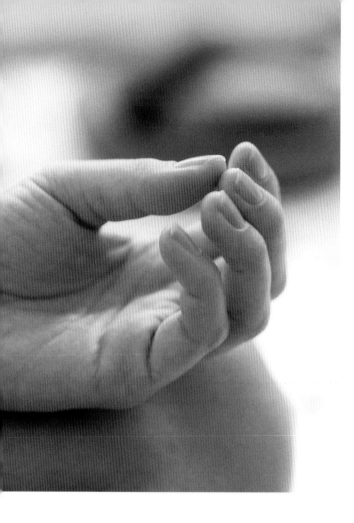

Meditation techniques

There are various meditation techniques you can use. Two alternatives are suggested below. Over the course of the weekend, you may want to try both to see if one seems more suitable than the other. However, normally you would give each one 10 days before you decide whether to try the alternative. When you have found a method you like, you should practice it regularly. Try to practice each session at the same time in the same place. When you become more adept, you will be able to meditate at any time in any place.

The breath

Close your eyes and be aware of your breathing. Count each breath, breathing fairly deeply, so that you feel your abdomen rise and fall. Inhale on one, exhale on two, inhale on three, and so on. Your breathing should be even, and you can focus the counting either on the sensation of the air entering through your nose, or the rise and fall of your abdomen. If you lose count – and you will – start again at one.

The mantra

This is the silent repetition of a word. It can be a word that has a special significance for you, such as "peace," or one that has a resonant sound; the best known of these is the word "om," pronounced "aum," and pronounced on a slow exhalation of breath. Your aim is to reach a stage where the sound and its resonance fill your mind.

After the allotted time, allow the focus of your meditation to fade away gently and bring your mind back to the present. Take some long, deep breaths and become aware of your body and its sensations, gradually becoming aware, too, of your surroundings and the noises around you. Finally, open your eyes, but remain still for a few more minutes.

You can establish your meditation routine during the course of the weekend – in the morning and in the evening – for the future. It will be particularly beneficial if you meditate after gentle exercise, but avoid practicing for at least an hour after a meal. If you find your sessions immediately beneficial, you can add an extra one during the course of the day.

Lunch and evening meals

There are several techniques and treatments that will aid relaxation of body and mind, and diet has an important part to play in this. While weight loss is not the purpose of this weekend, if your body is working overtime to digest rich food, it is going to be more difficult to slow down generally. Therefore, the aim of your diet for the weekend is that it should be light, nutritious and easy to digest. Your evening meal each night is a nourishing soup and the main meal of the day is eaten at lunchtime, when the body's digestive system is working most efficiently. If you don't think one bowl of soup will be enough for you, you can have a second serving, or eat a slice of whole-grain bread with it.

If you want a deep, restful night's sleep, you should eat neither too much nor too late in the evening. Don't be tempted to drink alcohol; although it makes you feel sleepy initially, it is a stimulant and may well break your sleep in the middle of the night. Tea and coffee are also stimulants, so avoid these as well. Instead, drink plenty of bottled or filtered water throughout the evening.

Try to eat no later than 8 pm and eat slowly, concentrating on your food while you eat – don't watch television or listen to the radio at the same time. This will give your body the chance to slow down.

Soups

You may want to make your soup before you have the meditation session on Friday, so you can eat it afterwards. You can prepare all the soup for the weekend in advance, so all you have to do is get it out of the fridge as you need it. All of the recipes here serve four, so you can share it or save it.

Vegetable stock

Most of the recipes here call for vegetable stock. You can buy bouillon powder or vegetable stock cubes, but making your own is simple.

3 potatoes, chopped
1 onion, chopped
2 leeks, chopped
2 celery sticks, chopped
2 carrots, chopped
1 head of fennel, chopped
handful of herbs such as
    parsley, thyme or bay
2 1/2 pints (1.5 liters) water
salt
pepper

1 Place the vegetables and herbs in a saucepan with the water. Season to taste. Bring to a boil and simmer for about 1 1/2 hours, skimming the surface regularly.

2 Strain the stock through a sieve and store in the refrigerator until required.

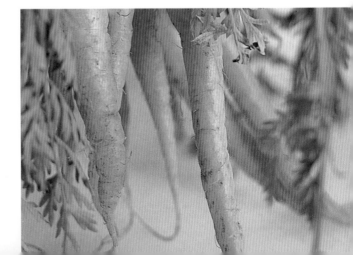

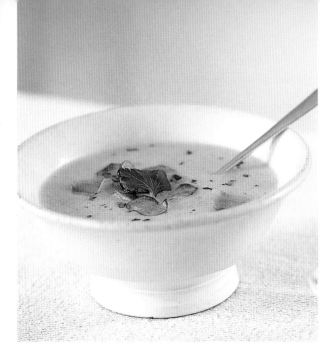

Jerusalem artichoke soup

Jerusalem artichokes have a delicious, nutty flavor, and make a particularly good soup, ideal for a cold winter's night. Garnish with lemon croutons.

1 lb (500 g) Jerusalem artichokes, chopped
3 tablespoons lemon juice
1 tablespoon sunflower oil
1 1/2 pints (900 ml) vegetable stock (see opposite)
1 teaspoon dried dill
1/2 teaspoon sugar
salt
pepper
Lemon croutons:
4 slices bread, crusts removed
1 tablespoon lemon juice

1 Sprinkle the artichokes with the lemon juice, then heat the oil in a saucepan and add the artichokes, stirring well. Cover and heat gently for 1–2 minutes. Pour in the stock and bring to a boil, then cover and simmer for about 30 minutes.

2 Purée the artichokes and stock in a food processor or blender with the dill and sugar, then push through a sieve and return to a clean pan. Reheat, seasoning with salt and pepper to taste.

4 To make the lemon croutons, brush both sides of the bread with lemon juice and toast until lightly colored on both sides. Cut into cubes. Serve the soup warm with the croutons.

Curried parsnip soup

This is another substantial soup that is particularly good for clearing any respiratory congestion. The sweet taste of the parsnips blends well with the warming effect of the curry. If you prefer a hotter flavor, add more curry powder.

12 oz (375 g) parsnips, scraped and chopped
1 onion, chopped
1 pint (600 ml) vegetable stock (see opposite)
1 teaspoon mild curry powder
1 tablespoon natural yogurt
salt
pepper
coriander leaves, chopped, to garnish

1 Place the parsnips and onion in a large saucepan with the stock and season with salt and pepper. Bring to a boil, cover and simmer for 20 minutes or until the parsnips are tender.

2 Remove from heat and allow to cool slightly, then purée in a blender or food processor, or press through a fine sieve. Stir in the curry powder.

3 Return the soup to a clean pan and reheat. Stir in the yogurt and serve garnished with chopped coriander.

Red lentil soup

This satisfying soup is a good choice if you are used to eating a large evening meal.

8 oz (250 g) split red lentils
1 leek, sliced
2 large carrots, sliced
1 celery stick, chopped
1 garlic clove, crushed
1 bay leaf
2 pints (1.2 liters) vegetable
    stock (see page 52)
1/2 teaspoon cayenne pepper
pepper

To garnish:
natural live yogurt
finely snipped chives

1 Place the soup ingredients in a large saucepan, bring to a boil, cover and simmer for 20–25 minutes or until the lentils and all the vegetables are tender.

2 Allow the soup to cool slightly, remove the bay leaf and purée the soup in a food processor or blender until it is smooth.

3 Reheat the soup, season with pepper to taste and serve warm. Garnish with a swirl of yogurt and the snipped chives.

Chilled celery soup

If the weather is warm, you might prefer this chilled soup. Flavorful and light, the cumin gives it a hint of richness.

8 oz (250 g) celery
2 pints (1.2 liters) vegetable
    stock (see page 52)
1 onion, chopped
8 oz (250 g) potatoes with
    skins left on, chopped
1 teaspoon ground cumin
3 tablespoons natural yogurt
salt
finely chopped celery leaves,
    to garnish

1 Thinly slice enough celery to fill two tablespoons. Set this aside and grate the remaining celery in a food processor or by hand.

2 Combine the grated celery, stock, onion, potatoes and cumin in a saucepan. Season with a pinch of salt. Bring to a boil, lower the heat and simmer, partially covered, for 20–25 minutes.

3 Purée the mixture in a blender or food processor until smooth, stir in the reserved sliced celery and allow to cool in a bowl. Chill in the refrigerator for at least 3 hours. Stir in the yogurt just before serving and garnish with the celery leaves.

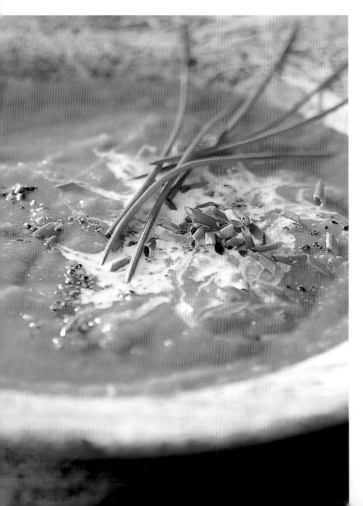

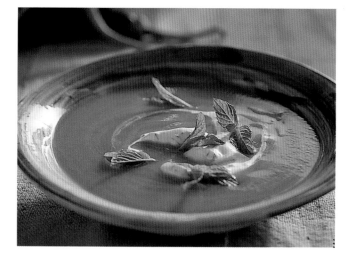

Grilled eggplant soup

Grilling the eggplants first gives this rich, delicious soup its distinctive, smoky flavor.

1½ lb (750 g) eggplants
3 tablespoons olive oil
1 onion, chopped
1 carrot, chopped
2 celery sticks, sliced
1 garlic clove, chopped
2 pints (1.2 liters) vegetable
   stock (see page 52)
2 tablespoons chopped basil
2 tablespoons Parmesan
   cheese, grated
4 fl oz (125 ml) natural
   yogurt
salt
pepper

1 Halve the eggplants lengthways and cook under a preheated broiler until charred and softened. Allow to cool, remove any charred patches and chop roughly.

2 In a large, heavy-based saucepan, heat the olive oil and add the onion, carrot, celery, garlic and eggplant. Cover and cook over a low heat for 15 minutes, stirring frequently, until the vegetables are softened.

3 Add the stock, bring the mixture to a boil, cover and simmer gently for 1 hour. Add the basil and allow to cool slightly.

4 Purée the mixture in a blender or food processor until it is very smooth. Return to the saucepan, stir in the Parmesan and yogurt and reheat gently without boiling. Season with salt and pepper to taste, and serve.

friday 9:00 pm **aromatherapy bath**

One of the most common manifestations of stress is insomnia, which can mean not being able to get to sleep or waking in the night and not being able to fall asleep again. Even if you do not suffer from insomnia, you may have a problem with light, restless sleep, which leaves you still feeling tired the next morning. This, in turn, can lead to tension headaches or general aches and pains.

One of the aims of this weekend is to have three deep, restful nights of sleep without recourse to medication and its unwanted side effects. Aromatherapy is a very pleasant alternative to sleeping pills and doesn't leave you feeling drowsy the next day.

You need to take time to wind down at the end of the day, which is why this first evening is so carefully planned, starting with the meditation. Eating a light meal fairly early in the evening also helps. If you feel thirsty later, drink a cup of herbal tea before bed. Chamomile with honey and lemon is ideal. If you have a tendency to indigestion, try peppermint.

Bathing

An aromatherapy bath is a very good way of slowing down the mind and relaxing the body at the end of the day. This is a bath that has little to do with washing; it is all about pleasure and relaxation. Prepare the room in advance to make it as tranquil as possible. The bathroom and towels should be warm. Lighting is also important; keep it as low as possible. Candlelight has a calming effect, and candles scented with relaxing oils are widely available.

Fill the bath with water. It should not be too hot or the oil will simply evaporate. Add five to ten drops of sweet dreams oil (see opposite) to the water and mix it in well. Relax in the bath for at least 20 minutes. If you have difficulty unwinding, listen to soft, tranquil music. After your bath, wrap yourself in a big, warm towel and pat yourself gently with the towel or just wrap yourself in it until it absorbs the water on your body, so that a little of the oil remains on your skin.

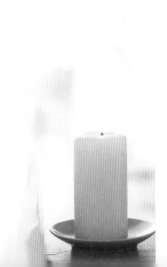

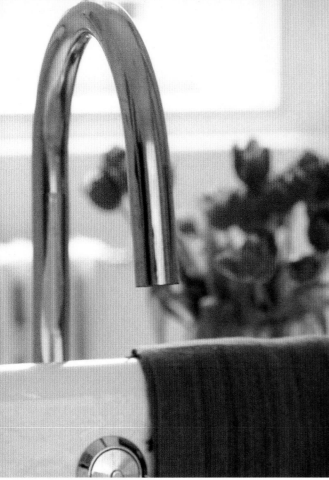

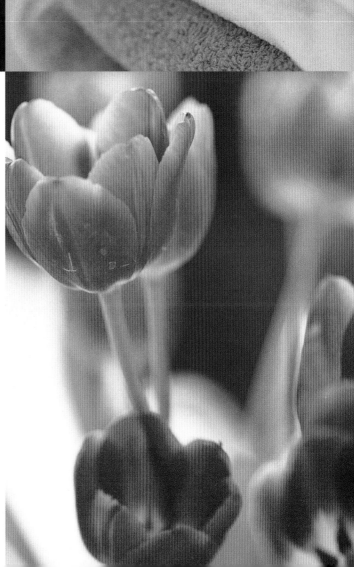

Sweet dreams oil

- 12 drops lavender essential oil
- 8 drops neroli essential oil
- 5 drops rose essential oil

Mix the ingredients and store in a glass bottle until use.

friday 10:00 pm **self-massage for sleep**

If you think you may still have trouble sleeping, there are several things you can try. Two or three drops of the sweet dreams oil (see page 57) on a tissue, placed on your pillow, may help you to unwind if your mind is spinning. If you still feel tense you can give yourself a facial massage. Use half of the mixture and add to it 1 oz (25 ml) of almond oil, grapeseed oil or any cold-pressed vegetable oil. Shake well and apply it to your face and neck. If you don't mind having oily hair until you shower in the morning, you can also massage the oil into your scalp. You should find this particularly relaxing. Alternatively, use undiluted lavender or neroli oil in a burner and put the burner in the bedroom about half an hour before you go to bed. Be sure to extinguish the burner before climbing into bed.

Self-massage for sleep

This self-massage, using the sweet dreams oil, will take you only about five to ten minutes, depending on how slowly you make the strokes. You can do it after your bath or even when you are already in bed, although in that case you will need a large pillow to support your back. Take your time and leave the oil on all night.

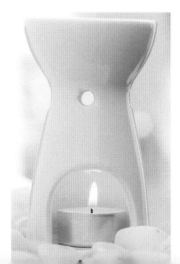

Facial massage

1 Rest your three central fingers of each hand on each eyebrow. Close your eyes lightly and remain in that position for a moment, taking a few deep breaths.

2 Place the middle finger of each hand either side of, and immediately above, the bridge of your nose, between your eyebrows. Now, following the line of the brows, make small circles with your fingers along the length of your brows as far as your temples. When you reach your temples, hold your fingers over them for a moment with a slightly increased pressure.

● Return to the center of the forehead, this time with your fingers placed very slightly higher, and trace another line out towards your temples in the same way.

3 Continue to repeat step 2, each time moving your fingers up slightly more until they are following the hairline. Then follow the hairline with the same circular movements all the way around to the nape of your neck. Repeat this several times.

4 Make the same circular movements from the neck hairline down your neck, with your fingers either side of your spine. Do not place them on the spine itself. You may want to use more pressure here.

5 Use the same movements from the center of your forehead back across your scalp to the nape of your neck. You may want to use two or three fingers here and make the movement cover a larger area. Finally, using the whole hand, cover the whole of your head, as if you are kneading your scalp.

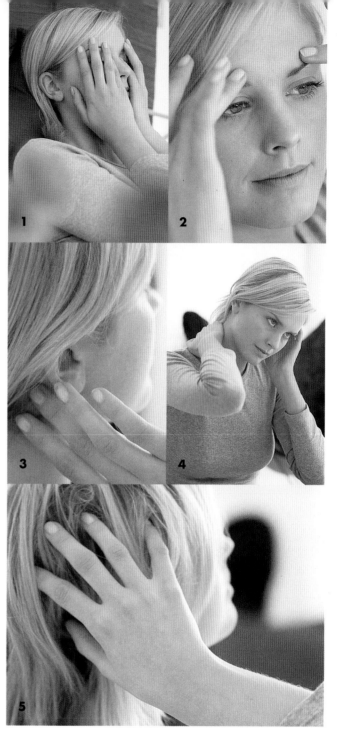

saturday

saturday 8:00 am **yoga**

Yoga, the ancient Indian "science of life," deals with physical, mental and spiritual health in its three disciplines of postures, or *asanas*, breathing exercises and meditation. During the course of this relaxation weekend, you will try all of these aspects of yoga.

Yoga is a systematic, gradual process of relaxation, and is therefore a perfect technique for this weekend. The physical relaxation that results from the practice of *asanas* and *pranayama* (see page 81) brings with it the release of old stored tensions, often emotional in origin. The body becomes much more supple, and the muscles become stretched and toned without increasing their bulk. Ailments connected with tension and contracted muscles are therefore often considerably relieved by yoga. These include chronic back pain, headaches and migraine. The effect of loosening immobile joints makes yoga particularly helpful for anyone who suffers from arthritis or rheumatism.

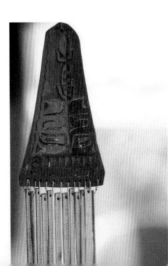

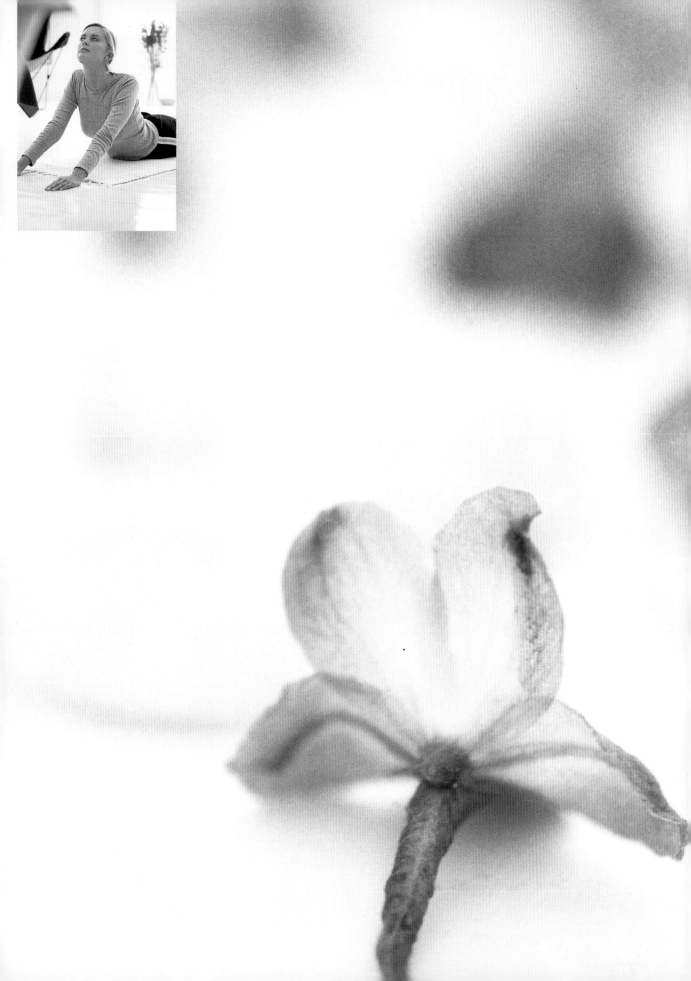

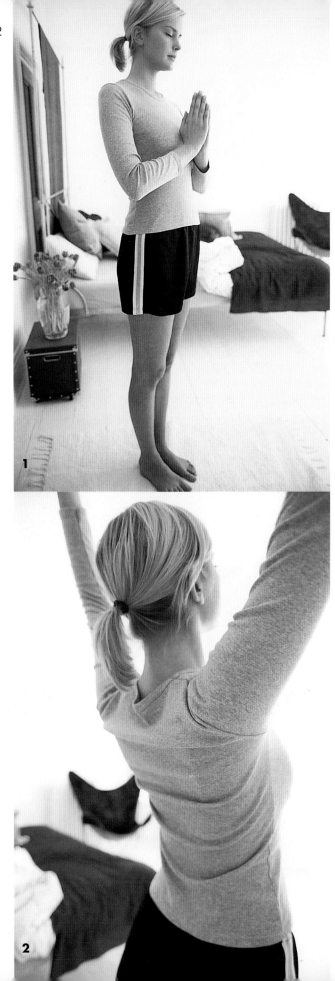

Start the day with the practice of a yoga exercise – before you breakfast or shower. Even if you are not at your best in the morning, this exercise will wake up your body and help to focus your mind. It also works as a massage for the internal organs. Wear loose clothing and make sure the room is warm before you start exercising – cold is not beneficial to stretching muscles. This exercise is called Salute to the Sun and is traditionally performed in the morning.

Salute to the sun

1 Stand up straight, looking straight ahead, palms together in the prayer position just in front of your breastbone. Check that you are balanced equally on both feet and you are not tensing any area of your body. Take a few long, deep breaths.

2 Breathe in deeply and stretch your arms up to the ceiling. Continue the movement so that your arms move slightly backwards, taking your body with them in a curve. Don't force this position any more than feels comfortable.

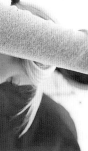

3 Return to the erect position, still with your arms raised above you and, as you breathe out, bend forwards from your hips, keeping your back straight.

4 Place your hands on the floor. If this isn't possible, hold the backs of your calves or ankles and gently stretch the backs of your legs.

5 Take a deep breath in and bend your left knee, at the same time stretching your right leg out behind you and placing your hands on the floor. Look up to the ceiling.

6 Breathing out, take your left leg back so that you are supported on your hands and feet and your body is in a long straight line.

7 Breathe in, drop your knees and chest to the floor as you breathe out. Keep your hips raised.

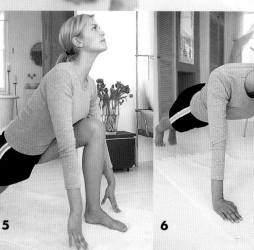

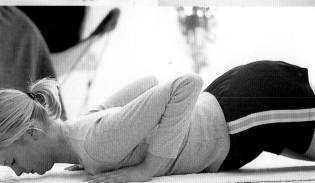

saturday 8:00 am
yoga

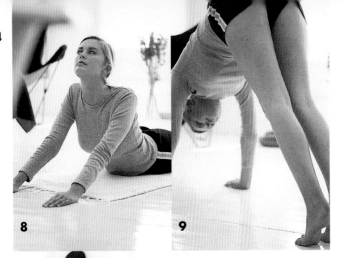

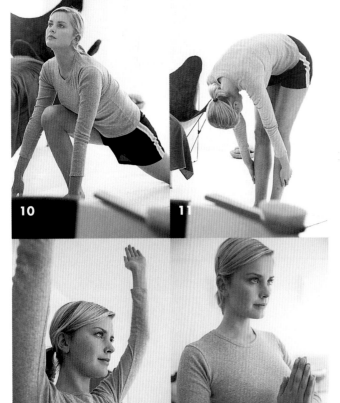

8 As you breathe in, drop your hips to the ground and in a long, snake-like movement, push your upper body through your arms as far as it will go until your back is arched and you are looking at the ceiling.

9 As you breathe out, lift your hips up to the ceiling and drop your head so that you make a triangle.

10 Breathe in, bringing your right knee forwards, leaving your left leg stretched out behind you. Breathe out and look up at the ceiling.

11 Breathe in and, as you breathe out, bring your left leg up to meet your right and stretch your legs, your hands flat on the floor or holding the backs of your calves. Keep your head dropped towards the floor. Only stretch as far as feels comfortable and, unless you are very supple, keep your knees bent.

12 Breathe in and very slowly start to lift your body from the waist, arms stretched out in front of you. Go past the upright position so that you lean back, arms behind you.

13 Return to standing and bring your palms together in the prayer position.

You can repeat this whole sequence a few times. Those who are experienced at yoga may do so up to 10 times. However, if you are a beginner, you should do it no more than two or three times at first. You will find that you can stretch a little further each time you do it.

You may also find it helpful to take one sequence very slowly, holding each of the 12 positions for a few moments and taking a few breaths to relax into them. When you have finished, take five minutes to relax in either of the following poses.

saturday 8:00 am **yoga**

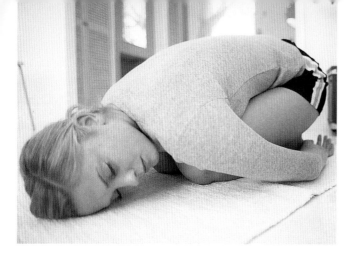

Pose of the child

This is a very good position to rest in after Salute to the Sun, particularly if your back is not used to so much stretching.

● Sit on your heels, back straight. Place your hands behind you on the soles of your feet. Breathe in and bend gently backwards, looking up.

● Breathe out and bend slowly forwards until you can place your forehead on the floor. You will have to let go of your feet, and your bottom may come up a little. Allow your arms to lie by your sides and breathe slowly with your eyes closed. After a minute or two of slow, deep breathing, allow your breathing to become shallower, but keep your eyes closed. When you are ready, come up very slowly.

Corpse pose

This is so relaxing that you might even fall asleep. Make sure you have something to cover yourself with in this position as otherwise you may begin to feel cold.

● Lie on your back with your arms slightly out from your sides with the palms facing the ceiling. Your legs should be slightly apart with relaxed feet. Close your eyes.

● Breathe slowly and deeply for one or two minutes, concentrating on the breath itself and the sensation of your lungs filling with air. Then breathe naturally for a few more minutes before getting up.

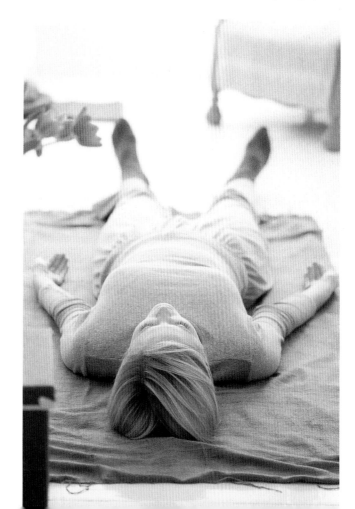

breakfasts

It is best to have breakfast after you have had your yoga session – exercise on a full stomach is not recommended. If you can, drink a herbal infusion rather than ordinary tea or coffee, but if you really can't do without these, try decaffeinated versions – you will sense the benefit when you do your relaxation session later in the morning, and when you go to bed at night. Drink plenty of filtered or bottled water or more herbal teas throughout the day and, if you want a snack, have a piece of fruit or some dried fruit and nuts.

Keep breakfast simple – perhaps a piece of whole-grain toast or a non-sugary cereal with some fruit and a herbal tea. Have a large glass of fruit juice as well – you could try making your own fresh juice (see page 22). The following are a few other breakfast ideas. (All of these recipes serve one.)

Figgy apple

1 large cooking apple
1 teaspoon clear honey
1 oz (25 g) dried figs
1 teaspoon lemon juice
1 tablespoon apple juice
3 tablespoons low-fat
    natural yogurt

1 Core the apple and stuff the center with the honey, figs and lemon juice.

2 Pour the apple juice and bake in the oven at 350°F (180°C) for 40 minutes.

3 Serve with the yogurt.

Hot fruit salad

This warm salad is also delicious when eaten cold.

4 oz (125 g) mixed dried fruit, such as apricots, prunes, apples, pears and figs
1/4 pint (150 ml) apple or orange juice
3 tablespoons low-fat natural yogurt

1 Place all the fruit in a bowl and add the juice. Leave to soak overnight.

2 Pour the contents into a saucepan and simmer gently for 10 minutes.

3 Serve with the yogurt.

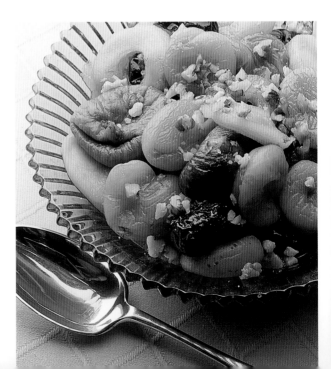

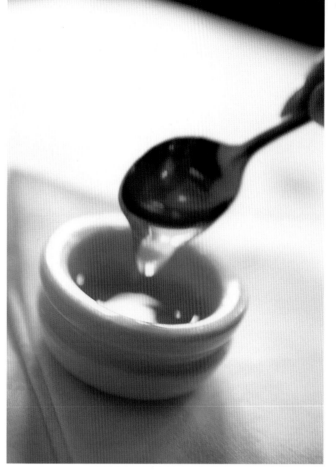

Melons with honey

1/4 small watermelon
1/4 small honeydew melon
1 tablespoon clear honey
1 oz (25 g) flaked almonds,
  toasted

1 Remove the seeds and
rind from the melons and cut
them into small cubes.

2 Gently stir the honey into
the melon cubes. Sprinkle
with almonds and serve.

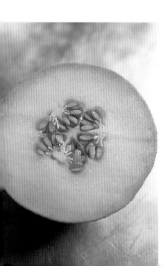

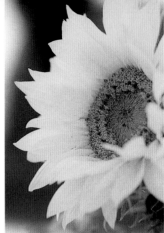

saturday 10:00 am **relaxation and meditation**

After breakfast, you can slowly begin to prepare yourself for the rest of the day, allowing yourself time to digest breakfast before you think about your next session.

Dress for the relaxation exercises in clothes that are loose and comfortable. Bear in mind that, during relaxation, your body temperature will drop, so make sure that you are going to be warm enough. Socks are a good idea and put a blanket or sweater nearby in case you begin to feel cold as the session progresses.

There are no secrets to relaxation, and when you try the exercises you may be surprised to find how closely the mind and body track each other. Where one leads, the other will follow; therefore by relaxing one, the other must also relax. However, you have to give yourself the chance to relax – free from interruption. Take the phone off the hook or put on the answer machine and, if anyone is likely to come in and disturb you, put a "keep out" notice on the door.

There are two ways of completing the relaxation process. You can either read through the instructions that follow and remember them, saying them to yourself in your mind, or you can record the whole sequence in advance. This allows you to focus entirely on your body.

Recording your relaxation tape

During relaxation, your mind and body slow down, so you must speak very slowly and calmly. As you will see, there is a good deal of repetition in what you say – this helps you to focus your mind. Leave pauses between each instruction – it is a good idea to take at least one long, deep breath between each sentence, with a longer pause between each individual instruction. In some places, for example where you have to repeat a series of procedures, you will have to leave enough of a pause for these on the tape.

You may not be able to focus on one part of your body immediately, and it is important to give yourself plenty of time. Don't put any modulation into your voice; it may sound boring to you as you record it, but you don't want any surprises or excitement during relaxation!

The whole tape, with pauses, should take 30–40 minutes, but you can take longer if you wish. You can estimate how long you need by reading the instructions aloud before you record them.

Some people like to play music in the background. However, this can be a distraction. You start listening to the music instead of focusing on your body. There are tapes available that feature music designed for relaxation and, when you have practiced the technique for a while, you may find one of these makes an interesting change.

There are many ways one can approach the relaxation process, and the one given here is very loosely based on the *yoga nidra* or relaxation technique. Nidra means "yogic sleep," but you are, in fact, very much aware, and carry your awareness around your body, focusing on each area in turn. Bearing this in mind, it is important not to fall asleep – so make sure the room is warm but not stuffy before you start. Put the tape within easy reach so you don't have to get up to switch it on after the preparation.

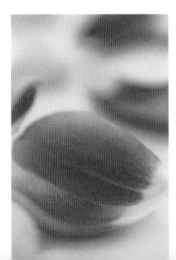

Preparing for relaxation

Lie on the floor in the Corpse Pose (see page 65),
covering yourself with a blanket or towel if you feel cold.
Take three long, slow, deep breaths, concentrating on the
exhalation so that your body feels quite empty before you
breathe in again. Starting at your toes, and working up
through your legs and body, tense each group of muscles
in turn, then relax them and move on to the next. Do not
expect your muscles to relax completely at this stage,
simply become aware of them. Some parts of your body,
such as your shoulders and your head, you will need to
move by rolling or rotating, rather than tensing. These are
all very slight movements. When you have become aware
of all parts of your body, simply lie still for a few
moments, still with legs slightly apart and hands by your
sides, and then switch on the tape.

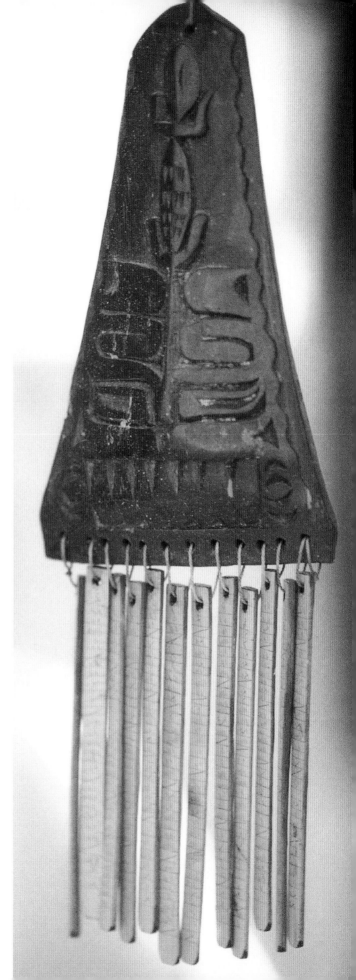

Relaxation exercise

Focus your awareness on your left foot. Become aware of your left foot. Take your awareness into your toes.

- Become aware of your big toe. Feel your big toe soften and relax. Become aware of your second toe. Feel it soften and relax. Become aware of your third toe. Feel it soften and relax. Become aware of your fourth toe. Feel it soften and relax. Become aware of your little toe. Feel it soften and relax. All your toes are soft and relaxed.
- Take your awareness into the sole of the foot. It is relaxing. Your left sole is relaxed.
- Take your awareness into your left heel. It is relaxing. Your left heel is relaxed.
- Take your awareness into the top of your foot. It is relaxing. The top of your foot is relaxed.
- Become aware of your left ankle. It is relaxing. Your left ankle is relaxed.
- Become aware of your left calf, the calf muscle, the shin, the knee. Your left calf is relaxing. It has become relaxed. The shin is relaxing. It has become relaxed. Your left knee is relaxing. It has become relaxed.
- Let your awareness flow up towards your thigh. Feel the muscles in the front of your thigh relaxing. They are relaxed.
- Feel the muscles in the back of your thigh relaxing. They are relaxed.
- Let your awareness travel higher, up into your left buttock. Feel your buttock muscles relaxing. They are relaxed.
- The whole of your left leg, from your toes to your buttocks, is now relaxed.

Now repeat the whole sequence on the right leg.

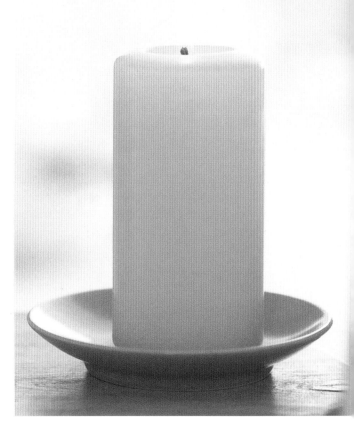

Take your awareness into your abdomen.

- Become aware of your abdomen. Become aware of how your abdomen rises and falls as you breathe. Become aware of the rising and falling. Your abdomen is relaxing. Your breathing is relaxing. Your abdomen is relaxed.
- Focus your awareness on your pelvic area. Become aware of the sexual organs, the bladder, the colon. Feel them all relaxing. The whole pelvic area is relaxed.
- Become aware of your back. Feel your lower back, your middle back, your upper back against the floor. Feel your lower back, your middle back, your upper back relaxing. Your whole back is relaxed.
- Become aware of your chest. Become aware of it rising and falling as you breathe. Feel your lungs expand and contract as you breathe. Feel your lungs soften and relax. Feel your chest soften and relax. The whole of your chest area is relaxed.

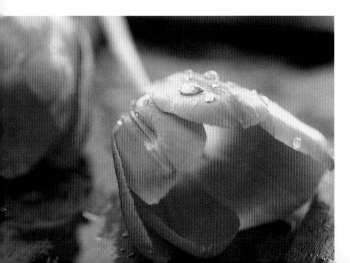

Take your awareness into your left hand.

- Become aware of your fingers. Become aware of your little finger. Feel it soften and relax. Become aware of your next finger. Feel it soften and relax. Become aware of your middle finger. Feel it soften and relax. Become aware of your index finger. Feel it soften and relax. Become aware of your thumb. Feel it soften and relax. All your fingers are relaxed.
- Become aware of your palm. Your palm is relaxing. It is relaxed.
- Become aware of the back of your hand. The back of your hand is relaxing. It is relaxed.
- Become aware of your wrist. Your wrist is relaxing. It is relaxed.
- Become aware of your forearm, front and back. It is relaxing. The whole of your forearm is relaxed.
- Become aware of your elbow. Your elbow is relaxing. It is relaxed.
- Become aware of your upper arm, front and back. It is relaxing. The whole of your upper arm is relaxed.
- Become aware of your left shoulder. It is relaxing. Your shoulder is relaxed. The whole of your left arm is relaxed.

Repeat on your right arm.

saturday 10:00 am
relaxation and meditation

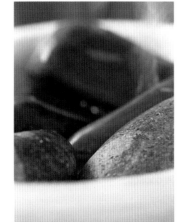

Take your awareness upwards to your neck.

- Become aware of your throat and neck. They are relaxing. Your throat and neck are relaxed.
- Become aware of your face. Become aware of your jaw, your chin, your cheeks, your nose, your lips. They are all relaxing. Inside your mouth, your tongue, your lips, all are relaxing. Become aware of your left eye, the eyelid, the eyebrow. They are all relaxing. Become aware of your right eye, the eyelid, the eyebrow. They are all relaxing. Become aware of your forehead. It is relaxing. Your forehead is relaxed. The whole of your face is relaxed.
- Become aware of your ears. Your ears are relaxing. They are relaxed.
- Become aware of your head, your scalp. The whole of your scalp is relaxing. The whole of your head is relaxed.
- Become aware of a point at the top of your head. It is relaxing. The top of your head is relaxed. The top of your head is opening like a flower.
- Golden light is pouring into the top of your head. It is pouring through your head, down through your body, through your arms, through your legs. The golden light is bringing peace and healing to your whole body. Be aware of your whole body pulsing with golden light.
- Feel the top of your head close, like a flower closing its petals for the night. The top of your head is closed but your body is still filled with golden light. Feel the golden light stream through your body on your breath. Feel how light and weightless your body is on the floor.
- Become aware of the lightness of your breath. Become aware of your breath coming into your body. Become aware of your breath leaving your body. Be aware of your breath for a few moments.
- Take your awareness into the rest of your body. Become aware of your arms, your legs, your back, your chest, your abdomen. Be aware of it breathing on the floor.

Completion

Lie on the floor for at least five minutes after the relaxation sequence. If you get up too soon, you may feel dizzy. Instead, lie on the floor, gradually coming back to your normal consciousness. You may want to lie on the bed for a while afterwards or even take a short nap. Do whatever you feel instinctively and spend the time until lunch as quietly as possible.

L

Lu
so
an
ea

G
ta

Se

½

½

6

½

8

2

wh

Tal

1 t

2 t

1 t

1 t

1 s

sal

pe

Hot chicken and walnut salad

Serves 1

2 oz (50 g) sugar snap
  peas, halved
4 oz (125 g) mixed salad
  leaves
½ red onion, thinly sliced
1 skinless chicken breast fillet
2 tablespoons olive oil
1 tablespoon walnut oil
1 garlic clove, crushed
1 tablespoon wine vinegar
1 oz (25 g) walnut pieces
pared rind of ½ lemon,
  thinly sliced
½ teaspoon soft light brown
  sugar
salt
pepper
parsley sprigs, roughly
  chopped, to garnish

1 Bring a saucepan of water
to a boil, add the sugar
snap peas and blanch for
1 minute. Drain thoroughly.

2 Tear the salad leaves into
bite-size pieces. Arrange on
a plate with the sugar snap
peas and the onion.

3 Cut the chicken breast into
thick slices. Using a rolling
pin, flatten the slices
between 2 sheets of
greaseproof paper or cling-
film to make thin medallions.

4 Heat the olive oil in a
frying pan or wok. Add the
chicken pieces, a few at a
time, and cook over a high
heat for about 2 minutes,
turning once, until lightly
browned and cooked
through.

5 Add the walnut oil to the
pan, stir in the remaining
ingredients and season with
salt and pepper. Heat
through, stirring, then return
the chicken to the pan.

6 Toss the chicken in just
enough of the hot dressing to
coat, then pile the chicken
mixture in the center of the
salad leaves. Garnish with
parsley and serve.

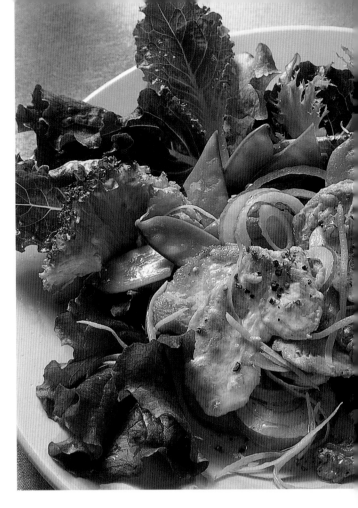

These delicious desserts are full of vitamin C, so you can treat yourself and know that you're doing your body good too.

Frozen yogurt with melon

Serves 4

large cantaloupe
1/2 pint (300 ml) low-fat
   natural yogurt

1 Halve the melon and scoop out all the seeds. Scoop the flesh into a food processor or blender and process until smooth.

2 Mix the melon purée with the yogurt.

3 Transfer to a shallow freezer container and freeze until firm.

4 Remove from the freezer about 20 minutes before serving. Serve in scoops.

Whole strawberry ice cream

Serves 4

3 egg yolks
1 tablespoon red currant jelly
1 tablespoon red vermouth
1/2 pint (300 ml) low-fat
   natural yogurt
12 oz (375 g) ripe
   strawberries, hulled
4–6 strawberries, with stalks,
   halved, to decorate

1 Put the egg yolks into a food processor or blender with the red currant jelly, red vermouth, yogurt and half the strawberries. Blend together until smooth.

2 Transfer the mixture to a shallow freezerproof container and freeze until the mixture starts to harden around the edges.

3 Tip the ice cream into a bowl and beat to break up the ice crystals. Chop all the remaining hulled strawberries and mix them into the ice cream. Return to the container and freeze until firm.

4 Remove the ice cream from the freezer about 20 minutes before serving. Serve in scoops, decorated with strawberry halves.

Spiced pears

Serves 4

4 large firm pears
1/2 lemon
16 cloves
1/2 cinnamon stick
1/2 pint (300 ml) apple juice
2 tablespoons red currant
   jelly
4 orange slices
4 small bay leaves, to
   decorate

1 Peel the pears, leaving the stalks intact. Rub them all over with the lemon half to prevent discoloration.

2 Stud each pear with four cloves. Stand them upright in a pan and add the cinnamon stick, apple juice and enough water just to cover the pears.

3 Bring to a boil and simmer gently until the pears are just tender. Leave to cool.

4 Put 2 tablespoons of the cooking liquid into a small pan with the red currant jelly. Bubble briskly for about 1 minute until the jelly has dissolved.

5 Place an orange slice on each plate. Drain the pears with a slotted spoon and sit one on top of each orange slice.

6 Spoon a little of the red currant glaze over each pear and decorate with a bay leaf.

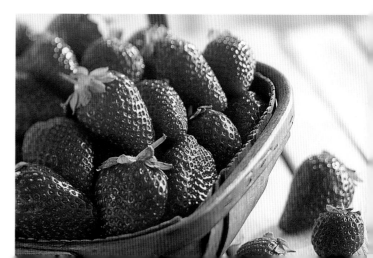

saturday 2:00 pm **massage**

Delay the massage until you have had a chance to digest your lunch. The ultimate treat is to have a professional massage – and it is particularly relaxing if aromatherapy oils are used. Look for a qualified therapist at your local gym, swimming pool or sports center, and make sure you book your appointment well in advance. Some therapists will even come to you. This is the best possible option; after you have had your massage you can simply relax at home. However, you don't need to find a professional. You can learn to give a massage very easily and, if you learn with a friend, you can take turns. There are a number of weekend courses available that will teach you the basics.

The massage described here is quite straightforward and very relaxing, particularly if you use oils. Oils will also help your hands slide smoothly over the skin, but always take time to warm them in your hands before you start. As with relaxation, it is important to keep warm, so make sure the room is warmer than you would normally have it, and that there are plenty of towels to cover up any parts of your body not being massaged. Cold muscles become tense, which defeats the whole point of the massage.

Make sure you aren't going to be disturbed and don't talk during the massage – unless it is to ask about the massage – as this is a disturbance in itself. When you give the massage, wear loose, comfortable clothes and take off any jewelry. You can either have a background of silence or play soothing music very quietly. Do the massage on the floor or a hard bed.

Try to trust your instincts when you give a massage and rely on your own sense of touch. You will soon get to know the feel of tense muscles that need to be released. Check at the start that you are using the right pressure for your partner – not so vigorous that it becomes painful or so light that it doesn't get to the root of the problem.

The body massage

The first person to be massaged should lie face down on the floor (with a towel underneath) or on a bed. Cover them with towels. In this massage attend to the upper body; it is the back, shoulders and neck that are usually the centers of tension, so you will be concentrating on the areas that need to relax most. However, you can continue and do a whole body massage if you wish. In this case, it is better if you start with the lower body and massage the legs first, then work up to the back, finishing, as here, with the neck and shoulders.

As the aim here is to get you or your partner to relax, you may find it most comfortable when lying face down to turn your head to one side. Turn your head during the massage or your neck may get tense on one side. Alternatively, you can put a pillow under your forehead to raise the head off the floor while maintaining a straight spine.

Never massage:
- Anyone with a heart condition
- Broken or infected skin or varicose veins
- Joints swollen by rheumatism or arthritis

1 Make sure your partner is lying comfortably face down and uncover the back. Warm the oil in your hands and place them flat on the lower back, with your fingers pointing towards the neck. Leave your hands still for a moment to let your partner get used to your touch.

● With your hands on either side of the spine – not on the spine itself – gently glide up the back, spreading the oil as you go.

2 When you get to the top of the back, move out to the shoulders and then gently along the sides. Repeat this several times, keeping your hands flat throughout, in a slow stroking movement. In massage technique, this is known as effleurage.

3 Starting again at the base of the spine, work up the back, with the hands either side of the spine. This time, make little circles, using your thumbs only. You can apply more pressure in this movement, and it is a very good way of releasing tension knots. However, check with your partner that you are not using too much pressure. It should not hurt.

● Repeat several times. Remember, never massage the spine itself. Always work to each side of it.

4 Knead the neck muscles, using both hands in the same way as you would knead bread. Knead gently here as these muscles can often be very tense.

5 Place one hand on top of the other at the neck. Make a figure of eight movement across the upper back, using the weight of your body to iron out the tension. Your hands circle the first shoulder, then move diagonally across the back to circle the opposite shoulder blade, returning to the center of the back and circling the first shoulder again. Repeat this several times.

6 Move around to your partner's head and, with your fingers pointing down the back, make a long stroking movement all the way down the back, placing your hands on either side of the spine. Use your body weight to help release tense muscles. At the base of the spine, move your hands out across the tops of the buttocks, then up the sides back to the shoulders. Repeat this step several times, gradually making the pressure lighter with each repetition.

7 Starting at the base of the spine, and using the middle finger of each hand in turn, stroke the whole length of the spine as far as the neck. Lift the finger off at the top and repeat with the middle finger of the other hand. Each time, the pressure becomes increasingly lighter, until it is as light as a feather.

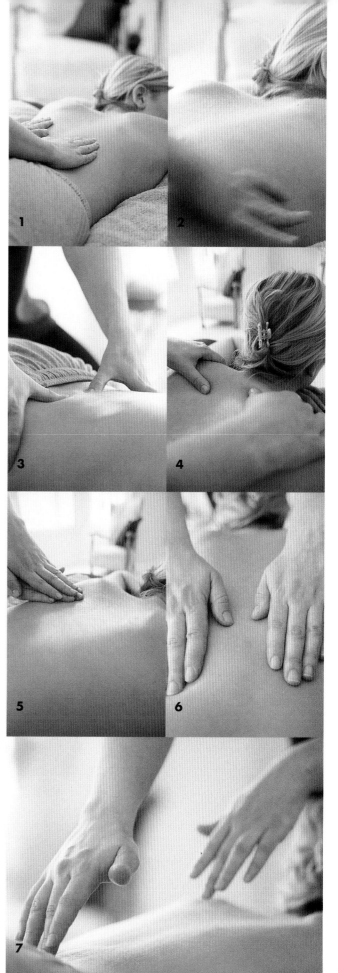

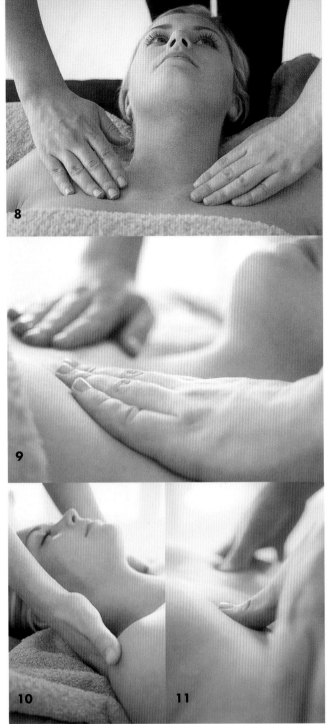

8 Ask your partner to turn over and cover them with towels, leaving the neck and shoulders uncovered. Warm some more of the oil in your hands. Lay them flat on each side of the upper chest and leave them there for a few moments.

9 With a long, firm, stroking movement, take your hands to the center of the chest, and then out to the sides.

10 Continue the stroking movements under the shoulders and back up to the neck, pulling out the muscles as you do so. This should help the back and neck to lie flatter on the floor.

11 Using the circular thumb movement you used on the back, move your hands across the upper chest. Start just below the collarbone, working outwards from the center. Repeat this several times, each time moving down gradually.

12 Place your hands, fingertips pointing downwards, on the upper chest. Move them out smoothly across the chest, over the upper arms, and up over the shoulders back to the chest. Repeat this several times. Place the hands on the upper chest and hold them there for a minute or two. Cover your partner with the towels and leave to relax for a few moments.

Relaxing massage oil

- 10 drops lavender essential oil
- 10 drops geranium essential oil
- 5 drops jasmine essential oil

Place the ingredients in 2 fl oz (50 ml) of carrier oil, such as almond, grapeseed, or any cold-pressed vegetable oil. Mix well and store in a dark glass bottle.

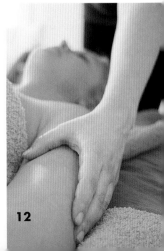

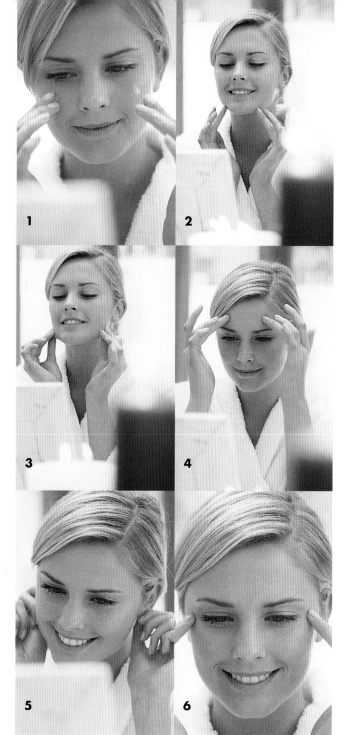

The facial

It may come as a surprise to realize that a lot of tension is stored in the muscles of the face. Frown lines are an obvious example, but rigid jaws, pursed lips and staring eyes are other telltale signs. A facial massage releases this tension and leaves your face looking relaxed, and therefore younger. Also, because the massage stimulates circulation to the face, your complexion should be toned and glowing by the end of this session.

1 Begin by cleansing your face thoroughly. Put on a light moisturizer, covering your throat and face with a thin layer.

2 Place your hands at your jawline so that your middle fingers are resting on your jaw, just below your ears. Making small circles with the middle fingers, work your way gradually to the center of your chin. Keep your jaw relaxed while you do this. Do this three times.

3 Return to the starting position, as described in step 2, but this time make gentle pinching movements along the length of the jawline. Repeat five times.

4 To release tension in your forehead, place your middle fingers between your eyebrows and make small circles as you work your way out along the eyebrows towards your temples. Repeat this several times, each time beginning a fraction higher up the forehead until you reach the hairline.

5 Hold your earlobes between your thumbs and forefingers. Gently rub the lobes between your fingers and thumbs. Now work your way along the outer edge of your ears, gently rubbing all the way, until you reach the top. Repeat five times.

6 To stimulate the eye area, begin with your middle fingers on the inner corners of each eyebrow. Now, making little tapping movements as you go, work your way along the eyebrow, then follow the eye socket round, across the top of your cheekbone and up the sides of your nose. Circle your eyes five times.

saturday 4:00 pm **facial massage**

7 Starting again at the inner corners of your eyebrows, squeeze along the whole length of the eyebrows using your thumbs and forefingers. Then move to your temples and, using your forefingers and middle fingers together, rub gently in a circular motion. Repeat five times.

8 Starting at the base of your nose, press your three middle fingers below your cheekbones, gradually working out in a line towards your ears.

9 Use all your fingers to pat your face gently in a ripple effect, tracing the outline of your face from your forehead, out past your ears to your jawline and into the center of your chin. Then let your fingers play over the whole of your face in a gentle tapping rhythm for two minutes.

10 Finally, rub the palms of your hands together and place them on your face so that the heels of your hands are resting on your cheekbones and your eyes are covered. Hold this position for two minutes.

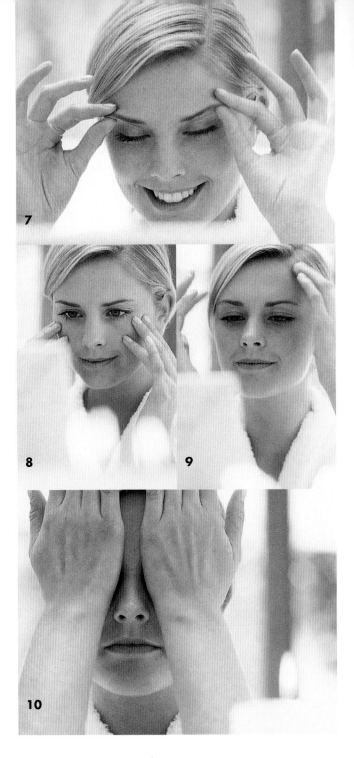

saturday 8:00 pm **breathing techniques and meditation**

Breathing relaxation

In yoga, ill health is regarded as the product of imbalances and blockages in the flow of energy, or *prana*, through the body. In this, it bears a great resemblance to the principle of *chi*, in Chinese medicine, such as acupuncture and acupressure. *Prana* is believed to permeate everything in the world around us and, in the human body, it flows in channels called *nadis*, which are equivalent to the meridians of Chinese medicine through which *chi* is thought to flow.

Pranayama, as its name suggests, is closely linked to the concept of *prana*. The practice of *pranayama* takes the form of breathing exercises. Unlike circulation or digestion, we can consciously control our breathing, and this acts as a link between the conscious and unconscious parts of our bodies.

Pranayama exercises improve oxygen intake, purification and circulation of the blood and lymph, increasing the flow of oxygen to every cell in the body. It is believed that these exercises also improve mental alertness, concentration and creativity, as well as being a form of deep relaxation, producing a sense of calm and serenity. Used at times of stress, when breathing typically becomes fast and shallow, they can dispel tension.

The *pranayama* breathing exercises, together with many of the *asanas* or yoga postures, also open the chest, strengthening the respiratory muscles and stretching out the lungs. This is beneficial for respiratory disorders such as sinusitis and hay fever, as well as asthma and bronchitis. Given the invigorating effect of improved circulation and posture, the body's immune system becomes more efficient, improving resistance to disease.

In both of the breathing exercises that follow, focus your attention on your breath and try to observe its progress through your body.

Meditation

The breathing exercises are very relaxing and slow the body down considerably. This puts you in the ideal state for meditation. So, as soon as you are ready, do your second meditation session, choosing one of the methods on page 51.

Deep breathing

This exercise helps establish a slower, deeper breathing rhythm, which in turn slows the heart rate and the pulse and aids relaxation.

1 Lie on the floor, placing your hands on your abdomen, fingertips touching. Take a long, slow breath in through your nose, counting to five. Your lungs and abdomen will expand, making your fingertips part.

2 Hold the deep breath for the count of five. Then, very slowly, this time on a count of 10, exhale through your mouth. Feel your fingertips touch again and keep on going, trying to empty your body completely of air. Repeat the whole sequence 10 times.

Alternate nostril breathing

For this exercise, sit comfortably on the floor, legs crossed, keeping your spine straight. Alternatively, kneel on the floor, sitting back on your heels, or sit on a chair. Choose whichever position is most comfortable for you.

1 Close your eyes and breathe in. Lift your right hand up so it is level with your face and, using your thumb, close your right nostril. Exhale slowly through your left nostril and then inhale again.

2 Now close your left nostril with the fourth and fifth fingers. Exhale and inhale through your right nostril. Repeat the whole sequence 10 times.

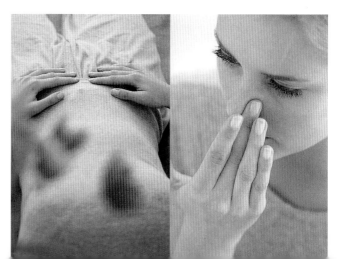

You should be feeling much more relaxed and well rested than you did when you woke up on Saturday. As yesterday, the day starts with a yoga session. Begin with Salute to the Sun on pages 62–64 – repeating between three and ten times, depending on how experienced you are and how fit and supple you feel. Then proceed to the following postures. As with all yoga exercises, do them slowly, and do not put any unnecessary strain on your body. If you feel at all uncomfortable or have any pain, come out of the posture, rest and then move on to something else.

sunday 8:00 am **yoga, relaxation and meditation**

Yoga postures

The following postures stretch, stimulate and bring into balance various parts of the body. The first, the triangle, involves a sideways bend that is beneficial to the spine and balances muscle groups.

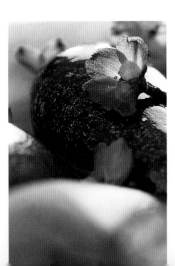

sunday

8:00 am
Yoga, relaxation and meditation

9:00 am
Breakfast

11:00 am
Acupressure

1:00 pm
Lunch

3:00 pm
Aromatherapy facial

4:00 pm
Meditation

6:00 pm
Evening meal

8:00 pm
Aromatherapy bath

10:00 pm
Bed

The triangle

1 Stand with your feet together, keeping your back stretched, and looking straight ahead. Your body should feel alert yet relaxed. Place your feet 60–90 cm (24–36 inches) apart, then turn your right foot so that it points outwards at a right angle to your body. Your left foot should point slightly to your right.

● Breathe in deeply and raise your arms to shoulder height, parallel to the floor. As you breathe out, bend to the right, placing your right hand on the thigh of your right leg, and sliding it down your calf as far as you can towards the floor. Do not twist your body as you slide down; your hips should be facing directly forwards.

2 Raise your left arm so that your fingers point to the ceiling and your palm faces forwards. Turn your head so you are looking up at your hand. Feel a long stretch down your left side and between your right and left hands. Take at least three long breaths in this position, 10 if you can. Breathing in, slide your right arm back up, dropping your left arm until you are facing forwards again. Repeat on the left. Do three stretches on each side.

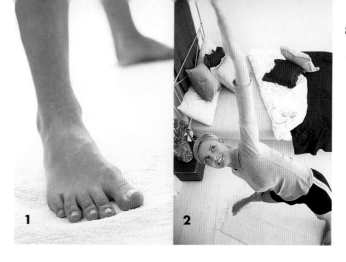

The cobra

The cobra stretches the front of the body and compresses the spine. The whole movement should be done slowly, with controlled movements, both while raising the body off the floor and coming down again.

1 Lie face down on the floor, legs together, toes pointing away from you. Place your hands flat on the floor, parallel with your chest. Your forehead should be touching the floor.

2 Breathe in deeply and slowly start to raise your head, feeling a stretch through the back of your neck. Look at the floor to avoid tension in your neck. Breathe out.

3 Breathe in again and continue to lift your head. As you do so your chest should come up from the floor. Bring your arms in front of you and use them to support your body as you lift the whole ribcage off the floor. Look directly in front of you. When you have lifted as high as you can without undue strain, press down on your hands, breathe out and, if you can, hold this position for several breaths.

● Breathe in deeply and return to the starting position, going through all the stages you did on the way up. Rest for a moment and repeat the sequence once more if you feel you can.

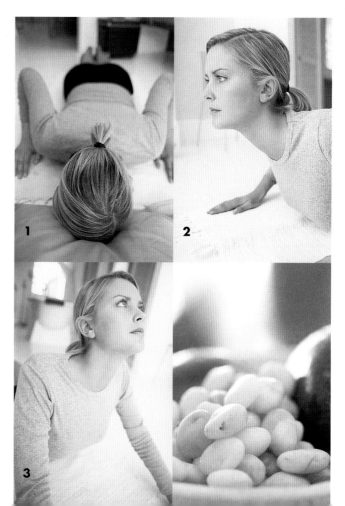

Shoulder stand and plough

The shoulder stand increases energy flow, improves the circulation and stimulates the thyroid gland. It also promotes body awareness. The plough is another inverted posture, or *asana*, that calms the mind but also stimulates the body.

Caution: Do not do the shoulder stand or plough if you are menstruating or have back problems. If you suffer from hypertension (high blood pressure) or neck problems, check with your doctor before trying these postures.

1 Lie on your back, arms by your sides, and breathe in as you bend your knees to your chest. Breathe out and straighten your legs as far as comfortable, taking them further back so your hips start to come off the floor.

2 Use your hands to support your back and push yourself a little higher. The aim is to straighten your legs so that they are completely perpendicular, while resting on your shoulders.

3 If you are able to get your legs into a vertical position, hold this position, breathing slowly, for one to three minutes. You can stretch and flex your feet in this position to help your legs relax.
● However, you may find this difficult at first and it may be more comfortable to leave them at a 45 degree angle to your body. If so, go on to step 4.

4 Take your legs over your head and, if you can, place your feet on the floor behind you, toes curled under and legs straight. This is the plough position.
● When you are secure in this position, place your arms behind you, flat on the floor. Take several deep breaths in this position.
● You can either return to the shoulder stand and go back to the floor by reversing the first two steps, continuing very slowly. Alternatively, roll your spine down slowly back to the floor from the plough position.

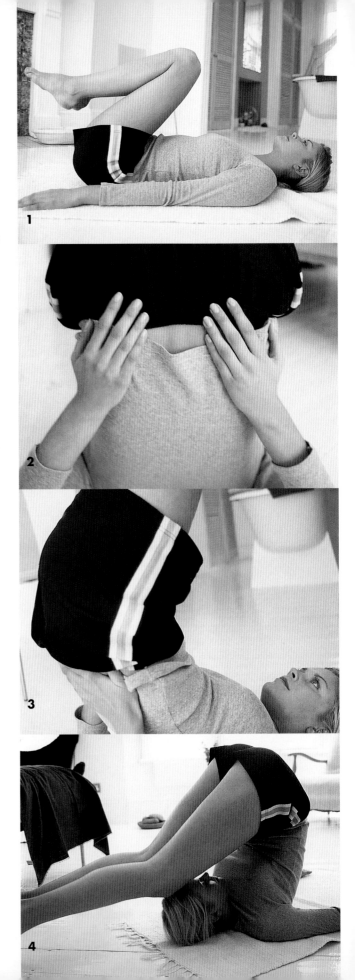

The fish

This posture opens the chest and compresses the vertebrae in the spine, so it acts as a counter position to the shoulder stand.

Caution: Do not do this exercise if you have neck problems. If you suffer from hypertension, avoid putting your head on the floor in step 2, as there is a vital pressure point at the top of the head. As an alternative, you can bend your head back until it is about 1 inch (2.5 cm) from the floor.

1 Lie on your back with your legs held together in front of you and your toes stretching away. Raise your back off the ground.

2 Arch your back, supporting yourself on your elbows with your lower arms flat on the floor, palms facing down. Lower the top of your head to the floor. Hold the position and take several deep breaths.

● Slide the back of your head and then your neck back down to the floor. Relax for a few moments.

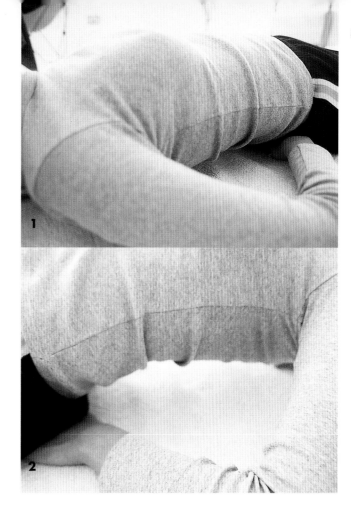

Relaxation and meditation

At the end of this longer yoga session, spend at least 5 minutes in one of the relaxation poses, either the corpse pose or the pose of the child (see page 65). You will now be in an ideal frame of mind for meditation. Meditate for up to 20 minutes and, if you wish, do the relaxation and meditation session (see pages 70–71).

sunday 8:00 am **yoga, relaxation and meditation**

Acupressure

Acupressure gives many of the benefits of acupuncture, with the great benefit that you can do it yourself, and no needles are involved. As with all forms of Chinese medicine, the underlying principle is that the smooth flow of the body's energy, or *chi*, is vital to health and well being. It travels around the body in channels known as meridians. If the energy flow is blocked as a result of physical or emotional disturbances, the body is thrown off balance. By restoring the flow of *chi*, health is restored.

Stress is all too likely to affect the flow of *chi*. It can result in many symptoms and ailments, including headaches, digestive upsets and insomnia.

sunday 11:00 am **acupressure**

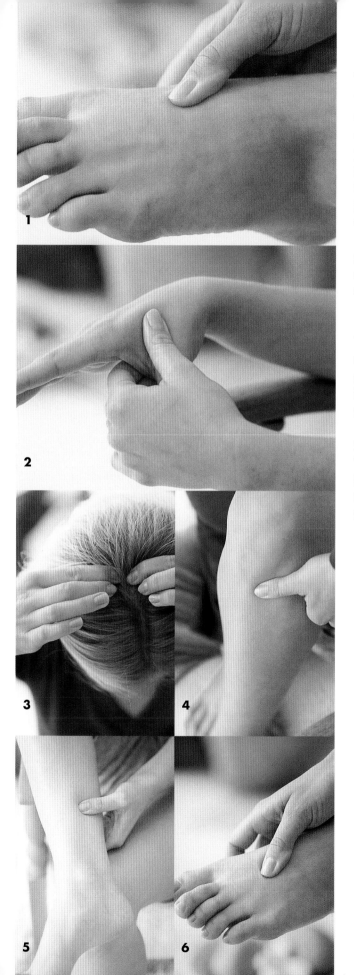

The right pressure

You can use your thumb or fingertip to apply pressure on a particular acupressure point. Use a firm, constant pressure with the finger or thumb held straight on the point. Keep the pressure even for two minutes.

There are two main pressure points for general stress relief, both of which are easy to locate yourself.

1 Foot pressure point

This is on the top of the foot, about halfway up. It is the point where the bones between the first and second toes meet.

2 Hand pressure point

This is located in the web between the thumb and forefinger on the back of the hand.

3 Head pressure point

This is the point at the center on the very top of the head. Caution: Do not put pressure on this point if you suffer from high blood pressure.

4 Headaches

The foot pressure point for general stress relief is good for headaches as well as stress. Another point is located four finger widths below the knee, outside the tibia.

5 Insomnia

The pressure point for insomnia is located four finger widths above the ankle bone, on the inside of the leg, close to the tibia. Caution: Never put pressure on this point during pregnancy.

6 Indigestion

This pressure point will help relieve heartburn and nausea. Find the point between the second and third toes, where the bones meet on the top of the foot.

Aromatherapy hair treatment

Before you start your facial, apply an aromatherapy treatment to your hair (see box). When you have made up the recipe, apply the mixture to your whole head, massaging well into your scalp and making sure that all of your hair is covered. Wrap a towel around your hair and continue with the facial. Leave the oils on for at least as long as the facial, although you could leave the treatment on overnight and wash your hair when you shower tomorrow morning.

sunday 3:00 pm aromatherapy facial

Cleansing masks

For dry skin:
Put 2 teaspoons of clear, runny honey in a bowl. Add 2 drops of lavender oil and 2 drops of rose. Blend well.

For normal to oily skin:
Put 2 teaspoons of natural yogurt in a bowl and add 2 drops of lemon oil and 2 drops of cypress oil. Blend well.

Facial toners

Pour 2 fl oz (50 ml) of bottled water into a small, clean mist sprayer.

For normal to dry skin:
Add 4 drops of lavender oil, 4 drops of rose oil and 2 drops of geranium. Shake well to mix.

For oily skin:
Add 4 drops of lavender, 4 drops of vetivert and 2 drops of bergamot. Shake well to mix. Spray over your face and throat with your eyes closed.

Essential oil skin conditioners

The recipe is for a larger quantity than you will need for just one application. The essential oils are blended in 2 fl oz (50 ml) of carrier oil. Use any cold-pressed vegetable oil or, if you have dry or problem skin, calendula or wheatgerm oil.

For dry skin:

Rose	10 drops
Lavender	10 drops
Sandalwood	5 drops

For normal to oily skin:

Lemon	10 drops
Lavender	10 drops
Cypress	5 drops

For mature skin:

Frankincense	10 drops
Neroli	10 drops
Rose	5 drops

Essential oil hair treatments

Add the following essential oils to 2 fl oz (50 ml) of vegetable oil.

For greasy hair:

Cedarwood	10 drops
Lavender	10 drops
Grapefruit	5 drops

For dry and damaged hair:

Rosewood	10 drops
Lavender	10 drops
Sandalwood	5 drops

1 Begin by cleansing your skin thoroughly. Use a cleanser that you remove with water. You can then exfoliate your skin with a mini-loofah, specifically designed for use on your face, while your skin is still wet. Use gentle, small circular movements, avoiding your eye area and concentrating on your forehead, nose, chin and cheeks. Rinse well with clean water.

2 Tone your skin with floral water. If you are using a proprietary brand, look for one that is alcohol free, as alcohol is not beneficial for the skin. You can make your own version very easily (see box opposite, facial toners).

3 Apply a cleansing mask to your face and throat, avoiding your eye area. Use any leftover mask on the backs of your hands. You can either buy a proprietary cleansing mask or make your own, according to skin type (see box opposite, cleansing masks).

● To make a compress for your eyes, put 1 drop of chamomile oil into 1¾ pints (1 liter) cold water. Mix well. Soak two cotton pads in this and squeeze out any excess liquid. Place over your eyes. Relax with the mask and compresses in place for 10 minutes. Rinse off with cool water.

4 Apply an essential oil skin conditioner (see box), according to skin type. You can use these as nighttime moisturizers on a regular basis, too. Apply the mixture to your face and throat. Leave it on for at least 20 minutes, then rinse off. Alternatively, you can leave this on while you are in the bath or all night. After your facial and hair treatment you should be feeling very relaxed. This is a perfect time for your evening meditation.

This facial deep cleanses and rejuvenates the skin. You can buy products over the counter that have essential oils added, or make those described here using aromatherapy oils and other natural ingredients. You may want to apply the treatments to both your hair and hands at the same time.

friday

7:00 pm
Autogenic training

7:30 pm
Evening meal

10:00 pm
Autogenic training

saturday

8:00 am
Autogenic training

8:30 am
Warm-up and stretches

9:30 am
High energy drink or muesli

10:00 am
Salt scrub

10:30 am
Aromatherapy

11:30 am
Autogenic training

12:00 pm
Lunch

3:00 pm
Ayurveda

5:00 pm
Autogenic training

6:00 pm
Evening meal

10:00 pm
Autogenic training

sunday

8:00 am
Autogenic training

8:30 am
Warm-up and stretches

9:30 am
High-energy drink or muesli

10:00 am
Shower (with optional salt scrub)

10:30 am
Reflexology

11:00 am
Autogenic training

12:00 pm
Lunch

3:00 pm
Chi kung

5:00 pm
Autogenic training

6:00 pm
Evening meal

10:00 pm
Autogenic training

The Weekend

This is the weekend for anyone who feels they are continually under par, performing at 80 percent or less of their full capacity. This weekend should be a tonic that puts you back on form, boosts your immune system and raises energy levels. If you wake up feeling tired and you would rather feel as if you were ready for anything, or if you are continually suffering from colds and the flu, and never feel completely healthy, help is at hand.

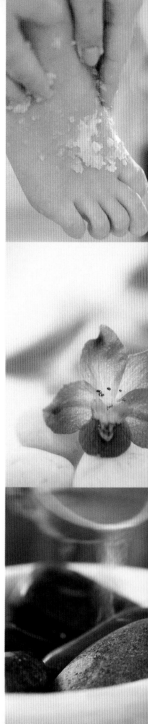
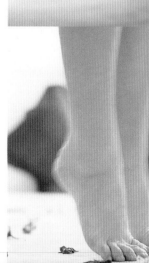

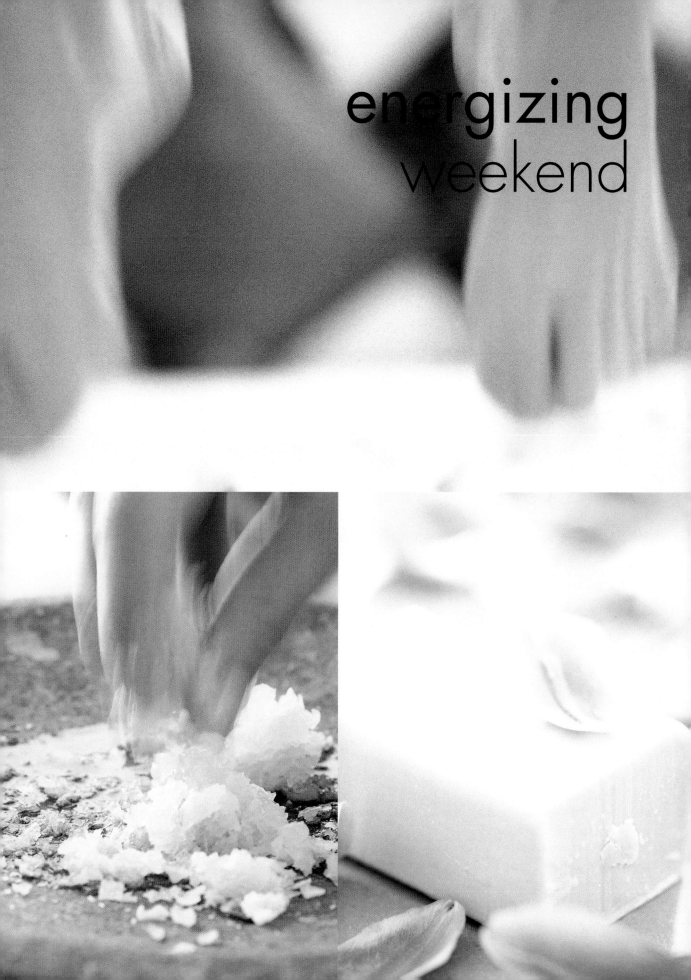

energizing
weekend

friday

friday 7:00 pm **autogenic training**

Autogenic training (AT) is a form of relaxation that verges on meditation. Stress undermines the immune system as much as pollution or a bad diet. AT is a technique that can be used both as a long-term relaxation therapy and also as a quick defuser of stressful situations. It is so easy and quick to do, it deserves to be a lot more popular.

Ideally, AT is a technique that should be learned with a therapist, who will take you through the several stages over a period of weeks. Unfortunately there are still relatively few AT teachers, so the bare bones of the technique are described here. You will probably find that you will not need to go any further than stage three during the course of the weekend, as the longer you spend on each stage, the more thoroughly you are likely to relax into it.

This is most definitely not a race. If you really feel that you are falling into a relaxed state very quickly at the start of each session, you could try proceeding to the next one, but it really does not matter if you find you are still on stage one by the end of the weekend.

Each session takes a matter of minutes. It becomes slightly longer at each stage. You can repeat each stage regularly throughout the weekend as you advance, but make sure you do at least four sessions a day. The best times are first thing in the morning, midmorning just before lunch, midafternoon just before supper, and last thing at night in bed. This is a very effective way of inducing a deep sleep. The minimum number and times of the sessions are given in the schedule.

You can sit or lie down during autogenic training. While you are learning the technique, it is a good idea to find a quiet room where you will not be disturbed. But, once you become more adept, you will find you can use it in all sorts of places and circumstances as an instant way of relieving stress – in the office, on a plane or before an interview.

As with all forms of meditation and relaxation, you should focus your mind quietly, without worrying if you find your mind drifting away on other thoughts. Just bring your mind gently back to where it is supposed to be. AT focuses on various parts of the body in turn and the sense of physical relaxation induces a mental relaxation. Focus your mind on the specific physical area at each stage. Don't worry if you don't feel heaviness initially – this will come. Don't worry either if you feel other physical sensations, such as numbness or floating. This is perfectly normal.

When you practice the technique in bed or on the floor, lie on your back with your arms at your sides, allowing your limbs to fall naturally. If you are sitting, make sure your back is well supported so that you can sit up straight, your feet flat on the floor and your hands resting on your thighs. Begin with a few quiet moments breathing slowly and deeply. When you have finished the session, sit quietly with your eyes closed for a few moments and gently bring your focus back to your surroundings.

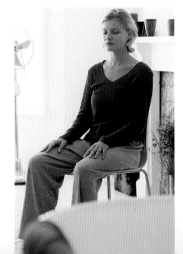

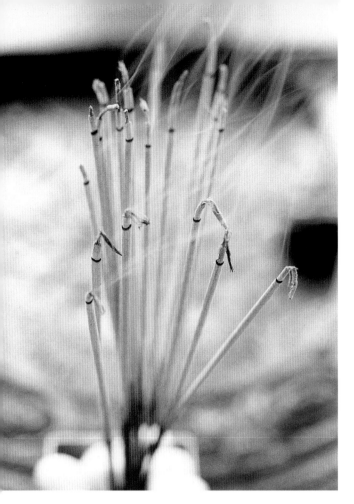

Stage 1

Close your eyes and repeat the following phrases silently to yourself three times each. Think the phrases very slowly and leave a pause before each repetition. Leave a longer pause before you begin the next phrase, so that your mind has time to refocus. If you are going at the right speed, it will take a minimum of three minutes, preferably closer to five to go through the following phrases. With each phrase let all your focus go to that part of the body.

- My right arm is heavy.
- My left arm is heavy.
- Both my arms are heavy.
- My right leg is heavy.
- My left leg is heavy.
- Both my legs are heavy.
- My arms and legs are heavy.

Stages 2–6 can be found on pages 122–125.

foods for strengthening the immune system

When you are under par in terms of energy, or are continually getting infections of one type or another, it may be that you have a weak immune system. There are a number of ways to strengthen the immune system. Of these, arguably the single most important factor is diet. There are certain nutrients your body requires to work efficiently and fight disease.

The World Health Organization (WHO) has now recognized the importance of the vitamins A, C and E as a means of fighting off disease, from minor infections to several forms of cancer – vitamins that most types of fast food do not provide in sufficient quantity. There are various other vitamins and minerals apart from these that are also essential to good health. Therefore, to maintain a healthy immune system, the advice is to eliminate, or cut down on, highly processed and high-fat food from your diet, and replace them with fresh natural produce, particularly fruit, vegetables and whole grains, and a little lean meat and fish.

The diet for this weekend concentrates on these foods. If you can incorporate some of these changes into your normal diet after the Energizing Weekend, you might find it helpful to follow it in a month's time with the Detoxing Weekend, and do another Energizing Weekend a further month after that.

The recipes on these pages are for all of the lunches and suppers this weekend. However, if you consider the fiber and fresh vegetable combination, you can make very quick snacks and suppers. One of the best is a simple mixed salad sandwich on whole-grain bread. Another excellent supper is a baked potato with a topping of hummus, served with a salad.

Supper should be a much lighter meal – soup or a baked potato is ideal. Breakfast is a high-energy drink and muesli; these recipes can be found on pages 104–105. Drink plenty of fluids – fresh fruit or vegetable juice, bottled or filtered water or herbal teas – at least 3 pints (1.8 liters) a day. You should avoid tea and coffee during this weekend.

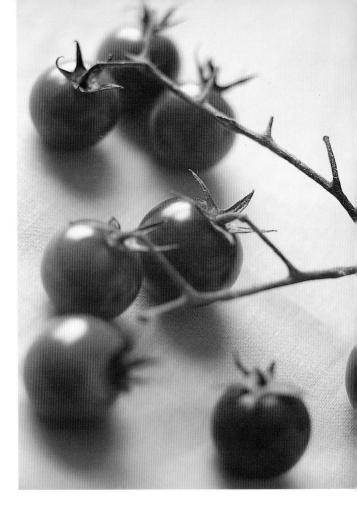

Foods for strengthening the immune system

Soups are particularly good in cold weather, as they are both nourishing and comforting. Another benefit is that you can make a large quantity and keep it in the freezer.

Zucchini and ginger soup

Serves 4

2 tablespoons olive oil
8 oz (250 g) onions, chopped
3 lb (1.5 kg) zucchini, thickly
   sliced
1¾ pints (1 liter) vegetable stock
1 tablespoon grated gingerroot
pinch of grated nutmeg
12 oz (375 g) potatoes, sliced
salt
pepper
¼ pint (150 ml) live natural
   yogurt, to serve

1 Warm the oil in a saucepan over a low heat and cook the onions until soft. Add the zucchini and cook for 5 minutes, stirring.

2 Add the stock, ginger and nutmeg and season with salt and pepper. Bring to a boil, add the potatoes and lower the heat. Simmer, partially covered, for 40–45 minutes.

4 Purée in a blender or food processor, return to the pan and reheat gently. Serve with spoonfuls of yogurt.

Lentil and tomato soup

Serves 4

14 oz (425 g) can plum
   tomatoes
2 tablespoons olive oil
1 large onion, chopped
4 oz (125 g) red lentils, rinsed
1 pint (600 ml) vegetable stock
salt
pepper
To garnish:
2 tablespoons live natural yogurt
handful of snipped chives

1 Drain the tomatoes and reserve the juice. Chop the tomatoes roughly.

2 Heat the oil in a saucepan and add the onion. Cook over a low heat until the onion is soft and golden. Stir in the lentils, stock, chopped tomatoes and reserved juice. Bring to a boil, stirring occasionally. Lower the heat, cover and simmer for 15 minutes.

3 Purée in a blender or food processor, return to the pan and season with salt and pepper. Heat gently and serve garnished with yogurt and chives.

Try to eat your main meal of the day at lunchtime, as this will give your body time to digest it before bed. A lighter meal such as a salad or some soup is ideal for supper. Whole grains are a good source of nutrients and fiber, so choose brown or basmati rice (with a little wild rice thrown in for flavor) and whole-grain pasta whenever you can.

Meat and poultry are a special treat, rather than a staple, this weekend. Make sure that you choose lean meat, organic if possible. Always try to buy fish fresh; many supermarkets now have a fresh fish counter. Eat fish within 24 hours of purchase.

Fresh fruit salad or a simple piece of fruit is a good way to follow every meal. Alternatively, you could try one of the dessert recipes on page 96.

Stuffed peppers

This recipe serves four, but if you are eating alone, you can make the same quantity of filling up to the end of step 2 and freeze the rest.

½ pint (300 ml) water
½ teaspoon salt
6 oz (175g) brown rice
4 tomatoes, skinned and chopped
1 onion, grated
1 oz (25 g) seedless raisins
3 oz (75 g) Cheddar cheese, grated
2 tablespoons chopped parsley
pinch of ground cinnamon
4 green or red peppers, cored and deseeded, with stem base reserved
5 tablespoons vegetable stock
pepper

1 Bring the water to a boil with the salt, add the rice and cook for 30 minutes, or according to the packet instructions, until the rice is tender and all the water has been absorbed.

2 Remove the cooked rice from the heat and gently stir in the tomatoes, onion and raisins. Stir in two-thirds of the Cheddar cheese, then the parsley and cinnamon. Season with pepper.

3 If necessary, cut a thin slice off the bottom of each pepper so that it will stand upright. Place the pepper on an ovenproof dish.

4 Divide the rice mixture equally among the peppers, sprinkle with the remaining cheese and cover with the reserved stem bases. Pour the stock around the peppers and cover with foil. Bake in a preheated oven at 400°F (200°C) for 30–40 minutes, until tender.

Tagliatelle with tomato sauce

This recipe serves six. For a single portion, just freeze the remainder of the sauce and adjust the tagliatelle accordingly.

2 tablespoons olive oil
2 onions, chopped
2 garlic cloves, crushed
1 lb (500 g) plum tomatoes, skinned and chopped
2 tablespoons tomato purée
4 fl oz (125 ml) vegetable stock
a few ripe olives, pitted and quartered
handful of torn basil leaves
8 oz (250 g) dried tagliatelle
salt
pepper
1 oz (25 g) Parmesan cheese shavings, to garnish (optional)

1 Heat half the olive oil in a large frying pan. Add the onions and garlic and sauté over a low heat until tender, stirring occasionally.

2 Add the tomatoes and tomato purée with the stock, stirring well. Cook over a gentle heat until the mixture is quite thick and reduced. Stir in the olives, basil and season with salt and pepper.

3 Meanwhile, add the tagliatelle to a large pan of boiling salted water. Boil rapidly until the tagliatelle is *al dente*.

4 Drain the tagliatelle, mix in the remaining olive oil and season well with pepper. Put the pasta on a plate, top with the tomato sauce and toss lightly. Serve sprinkled with Parmesan shavings, if desired.

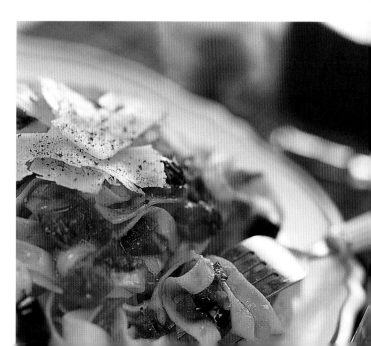

Warm duck and orange salad

This recipe serves one.

½ tablespoon olive oil
1 teaspoon sesame oil
1 boneless, skinless duck breast
1 zucchini, sliced
½ garlic clove, chopped
1 small orange, peeled and
    segmented
4 oz (125 g) salad leaves
1 recipe tarragon dressing
    (see potato and celery salad,
    page 39) using orange
    instead of lemon rind
salt
pepper
To garnish:
toasted sesame seeds
pared rind of ½ orange, cut
    into strips

1 Heat both oils in a large frying pan, add the duck and cook over a fairly high heat for 5–7 minutes, turning once, until well browned on the outside but still pink on the inside. Transfer to a plate, and keep warm.

2 Add the zucchini to the pan and stir in the garlic. Cook, stirring constantly, for 1–2 minutes. Transfer to a bowl and add the orange segments. Meanwhile, make the dressing.

3 Arrange the salad leaves on the plate. Slice the duck breast and arrange it next to the leaves with some of the zucchini and orange salad. Spoon the dressing over the salad and serve warm, garnished with sesame seeds and strips of orange rind.

Chicken tandoori

This recipe serves four. Halve or quarter the quantities if you want to serve two or one.

4 chicken breasts, skinned
1 garlic clove, crushed
1 tablespoon tandoori powder
½ pint (300 ml) low-fat natural
    yogurt
onion slices, to garnish
mixed salad, to serve

1 Make incisions in the chicken flesh and rub with garlic. Place the chicken in a large shallow bowl. Mix the tandoori powder with the yogurt and toss the chicken in the mixture. Place in the refrigerator to marinate for 3 hours.

2 Heat the grill to moderate. Remove the chicken from the marinade and place it on the grill rack. Grill for about 20 minutes, turning frequently and basting with the reserved marinade.

3 Transfer the chicken to a heated serving dish, garnish with onion slices and serve with a mixed salad.

Summer pudding

This pudding is enough to serve four. Alternatively, you can keep it in the fridge and have it on consecutive days.

8 oz (250 g) red currants
4 oz (125 g) black currants
4 oz (125 g) raspberries
4 oz (125 g) loganberries
4 oz (125 g) strawberries
4 oz (125 g) cherries or
    blackberries
1 tablespoon clear honey
margarine, for greasing
8 thick slices brown bread,
    crusts removed

1 Place all the fruit in a large saucepan (not aluminium or cast iron) with the honey and cook very gently for 2–3 minutes.

2 Line a lightly greased 2 pint (1.2 liter) pudding basin or mold with three-quarters of the bread, trimming slices to fit so that all the surfaces are completely covered and the base has an extra thick layer.

3 Spoon in all the fruit, reserving 2 tablespoons of the juice in case the bread is not completely colored by the fruit when the pudding is turned out. Cover with the remaining bread. Lay a plate or lid that will fit inside the rim of the bowl on top and place a 2 lb (1 kg) weight on top. Chill for 10–12 hours.

4 To serve, turn out and cut into wedges.

Spiced hot fruit

This recipe serves eight, but it will keep in the refrigerator for a few days and is good either as a dessert or as a breakfast. Serve with live natural yogurt.

3 oz (75 g) dried apricots
3 oz (75 g) dried peaches
2 oz (50 g) dried figs
2 oz (50 g) sultanas
300 ml (½ pint) apple juice
6 cloves
½ teaspoon grated gingerroot

1 Chop the apricots and peaches. Remove the stalks from the figs and chop. Put all the fruit into a bowl and cover with the apple juice and spices.

2 Place in the fridge and leave for 3–4 days, serving a bowlful at a time.

Monkfish salad

This recipe serves four.

1 lb (500 g) monkfish fillet,
  skinned
14 oz (425 g) can pimentos,
  drained
5 tablespoons olive oil
1 tablespoon coriander seeds,
  crushed
1 onion, sliced
2 garlic cloves, chopped
3 tablespoons capers, rinsed
  and drained
pared rind of 1/2 lemon, cut into
  thin strips
4 oz (125 g) mixed baby greens
Coriander and mint dressing:
handful coriander leaves, torn
handful mint leaves, torn
1 tablespoon balsamic vinegar
salt
pepper

1 Cut the fish into thin slices
and set aside. Rinse the
pimentos under cold running
water, drain well and pat
dry with paper towels. Cut
them into strips.

2 Heat the oil in a frying
pan. Add the coriander
seeds and cook over a low
heat for a few seconds. Then
add the onion and cook for
about 5 minutes, stirring
frequently until soft but not
browned. Add the garlic
and cook for 1 minute more.

3 Increase the heat slightly
and add the fish to the pan.
Cook, stirring gently, for
3–4 minutes, or until the fish
is firm and opaque.

4 Lower the heat, stir in the
pimento, capers and lemon

rind. Remove the pan from
the heat and allow to cool
for a few minutes. Remove
the monkfish and set aside.

5 To make the dressing, add
the coriander and mint to the
liquid in the pan. Add the
balsamic vinegar and season
with salt and pepper to taste
and stir.

6 Serve the fish on a bed of
mixed baby greens, drizzled
with the dressing.

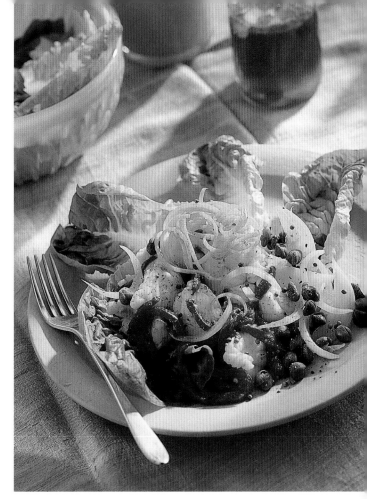

Tuna steaks with avocado

This recipe serves two.

2 tablespoons olive oil
2 tuna steaks
1 teaspoon chopped chives, to
  garnish
mixed salad leaves, to serve
Avocado dressing:
1 ripe avocado, peeled and
  pitted
3 tablespoons live natural yogurt
1 teaspoon lemon juice

1 Heat the oil in a frying
pan and cook the tuna
steaks gently, turning
frequently, until they are
cooked all the way through.
Remove from the heat.

2 Meanwhile, make the
dressing. Mash the avocado
in a bowl with a fork. Mix in
the yogurt and lemon juice.

3 Transfer the tuna to serving
plates and place a spoonful
of the mixture over each fish.
Garnish with chives and
serve with a mixed salad.

saturday

8:00 am Autogenic training	**11:30 am** Autogenic training
8:30 am Warm-up exercises and stretches	**12:00 pm** Lunch
9:30 am High-energy drink or muesli	**3:00 pm** Ayurveda
10:00 am Salt scrub	**5:00 pm** Autogenic training
10:30 am Aromatherapy	**6:00 pm** Evening meal
	10:00 pm Autogenic training

saturday 8:30 am
warm-up exercises and stretches

As soon as you wake up this morning, make yourself a cup of herbal tea. It will rehydrate you and set you up for the day. The exercises you do each morning after your AT session are based on stretching, which warms up and energizes the body. If you wish, you can leave it at this. However, if you are used to regular exercise, simply do the warm-up first and then continue with your usual form of exercise. Do the stretches after your exercise. Don't tire yourself out by trying to do more than usual. This weekend is about building more energy than you are expending. Brisk walking is a very good way of exercising. So is rebounding on a mini-trampoline, which gives a tremendous boost to the system, as well as being fun.

Ideally, do the warm-up before and the stretches after the aerobic exercise, when your body will be warmer and you will get a better stretch. For the aerobic exercise, brisk walking is ideal. Walk for at least 20 minutes.

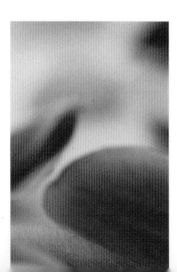

Arm stretches

1 Stand with a good posture, shoulders relaxed, back straight and navel gently drawn to your spine. Place your feet hip-width apart.

2 Stretch your left arm straight up to the ceiling. Bend your left knee at the same time, feeling the stretch all the way up your side.

● Repeat the stretch on the right side. Do 10 stretches on each side.

● Stretch your arms in the same way as before, but this time take your arms out to shoulder level.

● Alternate, doing 10 stretches on each side.

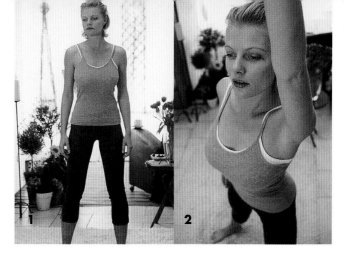

Shoulder looseners

1 Stand in the same position as you did for the arm stretches. Slowly roll your shoulders forward towards your chest. Keep your arms relaxed; they will move of their own accord.

2 Lift your shoulders up towards your ears and then move them towards your back, gently squeezing your shoulder blades together. Drop your shoulders back into their natural position. Repeat the exercise three more times, then reverse the direction and do another four.

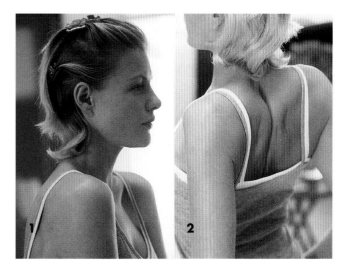

Waist twists

1 Stand in the same position as you did for the arm stretches. Fold your arms loosely in front of you so they are about level with your breastbone.

2 Turn to the right from your waist only. Your hips should remain facing squarely to the front. Return to the center and repeat to the left. Alternate, twisting 10 times to each side.

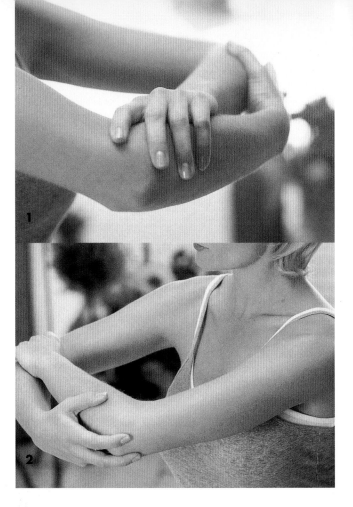

Side bends

1 Stand as before, with your arms hanging loosely at your sides. Now place your left hand on your hip and raise your right arm.

2 Stretch over to the left, feeling the stretch all the way up the right side of your body.
● Return to the center and do 8 more stretches on the same side, then repeat on the other side.

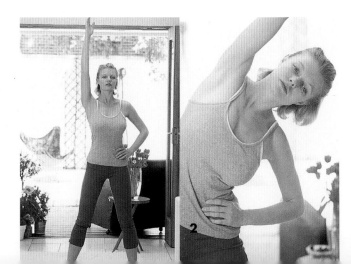

Leg swings

1 Stand up straight, feet together at the heels and slightly apart at the toes. Hold on to a chair back with your right hand, if necessary. Lift your left leg and swing it forward.

2 Now swing your leg backwards. Continue swinging your leg backwards and forwards so that your leg is moving in a relaxed way in the hip socket. The hip itself, as well as the upper body, should remain erect and still. You may find it easier to balance if you hold your left arm out just below shoulder level. Do 10 swings, then repeat on your other leg.

This is the end of the warm-up exercises and the point at which you should have some aerobic exercise. Brisk walking is ideal. Walk for at least 20 minutes.

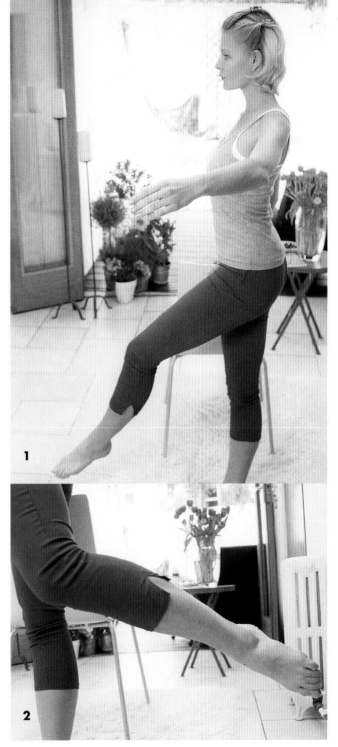

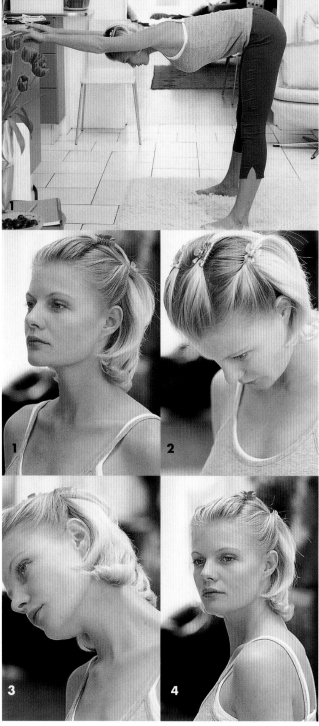

Depending on how used you are to exercise, take these stretches as far as feels comfortable. But don't overdo either the extent of the stretch or the repetitions.

Back stretch

1 Stand with a straight back, navel drawn lightly to your spine, your shoulders dropped down and feet hip-width apart. Bend forwards from your waist and rest your fingertips on the back of a chair or table. You should just be able to reach it and feel a long stretch in your back. Don't tense your shoulders. Make your back as flat as a table top.

Head rolls

1 Stand up straight, with relaxed shoulders, arms by your sides, feet hip-width apart. If you can, do this in front of a mirror. Look straight ahead so you are looking into your own eyes.

2 Now drop your chin onto your chest and feel the stretch up the back of your neck. Hold this position for a moment and try to relax into it.

3 Without tensing or moving your shoulders, roll your head towards your right shoulder. Then take it back to the center and roll it to the left. Alternate the direction, stretching your neck four times on each side.

4 Now lift your head again so you are looking straight ahead. This time, turn your head so that you are looking over your left shoulder. Hold this position for a moment, then turn to the right. Stretch each side four times, holding the turned position for a moment each time.

Leg lifts

1 Lie on the floor, with your arms at your sides, legs together. Check you are not tensing any part of your body. Lift your right leg straight up, toes pointing at the ceiling. If you are flexible you can draw it down further, towards your body; use a scarf looped round your ankle, if you like.

● Don't try to stretch any further than feels comfortable. Hold the stretch for 1–2 minutes and try to relax into it – your leg will slowly drop down further. Repeat with your left leg.

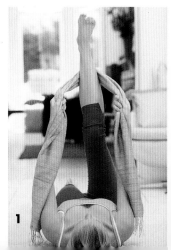

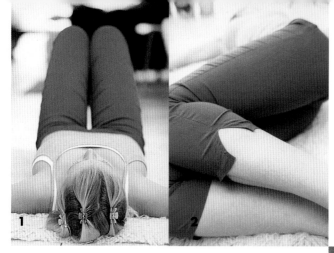

Diagonal stretch

1 Lie on the floor as in the last exercise, but with your arms out at shoulder level. Bend your legs so your feet are flat on the floor and your knees are pointing towards the ceiling.

2 Drop your knees down to the right and, at the same time, turn your head to look to the left. Try to keep your shoulders on the floor. You should feel a strong diagonal stretch across your body. Hold this position for a minute. Return your knees to the center and drop them to the left, turning your head to the right. Alternate four times on each side, holding the stretch each time.

The cat

This is a yoga posture that stretches the spine, promoting strength and flexibility.

1 Kneel on the floor, hands in front, to make a table shape. Your back should be as flat as you can make it and your head in line with your back.

2 Draw your navel to your spine and arch your back upwards, dropping your head down. Iron out your back so that it is flat again. If you have back problems, do only these two stages, repeating four times. If not, go on to the next step.

3 Slowly lift your head and push your buttocks up towards the ceiling so that your back forms a concave arch. Look up at the ceiling if you can. Return to the starting position and repeat the whole sequence four more times.

saturday 8:30 am
warm-up exercises and stretches

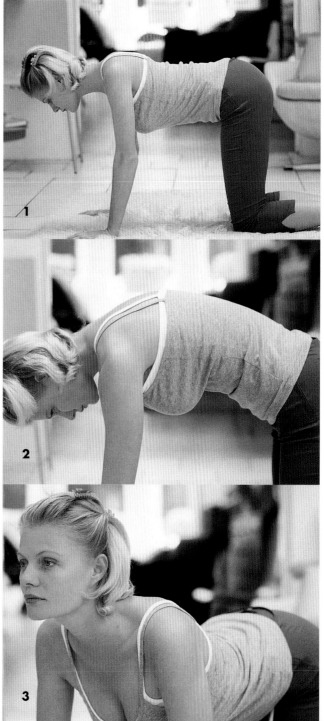

This weekend, you can have either have muesli for breakfast (see opposite) or a high-energy drink (see below). The drink includes live yogurt, which is good for the digestive system; the fruit and honey give you an immediate boost and go on to release energy throughout the morning.

You can vary the flavor of your shake on a daily basis, simply by changing the fruit. For the sake of sweetness, put in a ripe banana. This makes a delicious drink on its own, but you can then add all other fruit as well. Choose fleshy fruits for a rich, exotic flavor – peaches, apricots, papaya and mango

are good for this. For a sharper, fresher taste, try strawberries or raspberries. Very acidic fruits do not really work, but fresh, grated coconut is wonderful.

Try to avoid caffeine this weekend, if you can. If you absolutely must have coffee, have one small cup now, not later in the day. It does give you a boost, but it is a false surge of energy, and eating or drinking your breakfast is a much healthier way to energize. Instead of coffee, have a glass of fresh fruit juice or a herbal tea.

Drink plenty of water throughout the day – at least 3 pints (1.8 liters) – but only drink filtered or bottled water.

saturday 9:30 am
high-energy drink or muesli

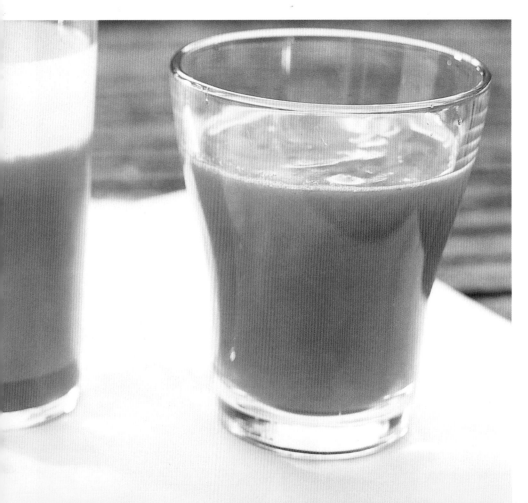

Yogurt shake

Serves 1.

large glass of live natural
    yogurt
1 teaspoon honey (up to a
    tablespoon if you have a
    very sweet tooth)
fruit, such as banana,
    peach, mango and
    strawberries

1 Put all of the shake ingredients in a blender and mix thoroughly.

2 Pour out and drink.

Muesli

This recipe is based on the original version, created by Dr. Max Bircher-Benner, a remarkable Swiss physician who made it a staple at his spa. You can add other fruit to the basic recipe: banana is delicious, thinly sliced. All the summer berries give it a fresh flavor, or you can use soaked dried fruit, which makes it a very rich, substantial meal.

2 tablespoons porridge oats
2 tablespoons raisins or
    sultanas
4 tablespoons apple or
    pineapple juice
1 apple or pear
1 tablespoon chopped,
    mixed nuts
1/2 teaspoon ground ginger
1 teaspoon honey (optional)
2 tablespoons live natural
    yogurt

1 Soak the oats and raisins or sultanas in the apple or pineapple juice overnight.

2 Next morning, grate the apple or pear and mix into the oats together with the mixed nuts and ginger and, if you have a very sweet tooth, the honey.

3 Pour the yogurt on top of the muesli and serve.

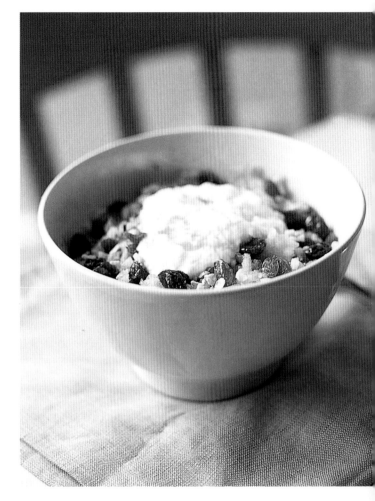

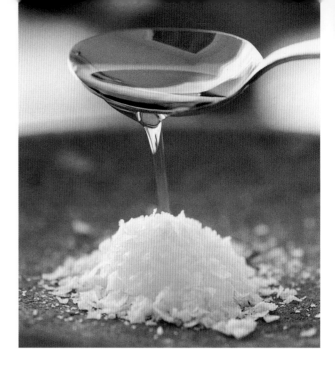

This is a gentler version of a treatment found in many European health spas, yet it is still guaranteed to start your day with a boost of energy. A salt body scrub has a number of beneficial effects, all of them stimulating to the system.

- It clears the pores, sloughs away dead skin cells, so your skin is fresher and smoother.
- It also stimulates the circulation and the elimination of toxins through the lymphatic system.
- It stimulates cell renewal.
- It will make your skin tingle and glow with vital energy.

saturday 10:00 am **salt scrub**

Preparing the salt scrub

There are many exfoliants on the market, yet one of the best is simple salt. You should use rock salt in flakes rather than fine salt (except on the face, see below). You can apply it directly to your body in handfuls, but it is easier to work with if you mix it into a paste with olive or sesame oil. This has the added advantage of nourishing the skin at the same time. You will need a handful of coarse rock salt and two tablespoons of olive or sesame oil. If you would like a slightly less functional smell, add one drop only of rose or lavender essential oil. Mix all the ingredients together in a bowl and take this with you into the bathroom. Make sure that the bathroom is warm and that you have plenty of warm towels and a warm, soft robe nearby.

Before you start your body scrub, you should exfoliate your face and neck. For this, you will need to make up a separate mixture, using fine salt, as rock salt will be too coarse for the delicate skin of the face. Use oil even if you have oily skin.

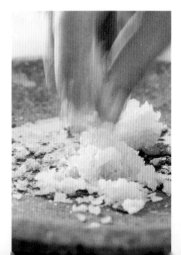

Face scrub

1 Using a face cloth, wet your face and throat with warm water. While it is still wet, massage the scrub mixture into your skin, starting from your throat. Use the first two fingers of each hand to make small circular movements from the base of your throat up to your jaw. Start at the center and work gradually along the sides.

● Apply the scrub mixture over your whole face, except for your eye area. Using the same small circular movements, work along your jaw line from your chin up to your ears.

2 Next, using only the forefinger of each hand, make tiny circles, starting from between your eyebrows, and moving straight up to your hairline; follow your hairline out to your temples. Repeat this from the center out along the middle of your brow and finally along a line just above your eyebrows out to your temples.

● Again, using only your forefingers, exfoliate down the length of your nose and out to the sides, then circle up to the starting point. Repeat this three times. Then, starting just below your nose, work out along the edge of your upper lip and then down below your lower lip, and over your whole chin area. Finally, using the first two fingers of each hand again, exfoliate your cheeks. Start on your cheekbones, working out from your nose

towards your ears. Repeat, each time dropping your fingers to a slightly lower starting point until the whole face has been exfoliated.

3 Rinse off the salt mixture by splashing lukewarm water over your face, which should now be soft and glowing.

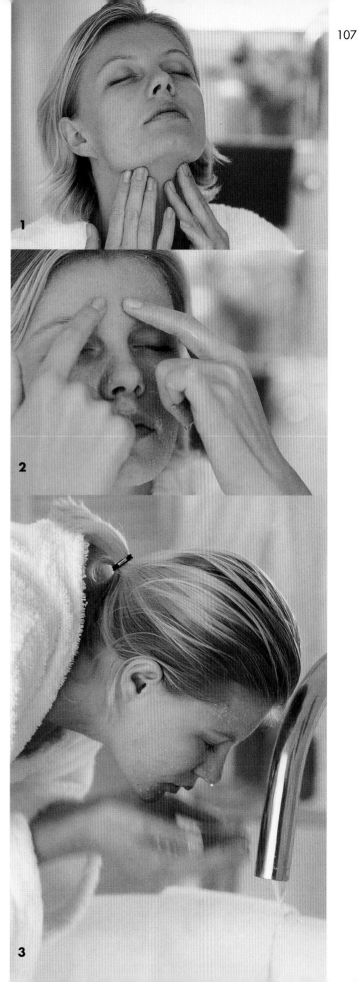

Body scrub

1 Stand under a warm shower for 1–2 minutes and make sure your whole body is wet. Step out from under the water, scoop some of the scrub mixture into your hand and, starting from your feet, massage it well into your skin, using circular movements with your whole hand. Make sure you scrub the soles of your feet, too.

2 Gradually move up your legs, using circular movements all the way. Pay particular attention to your thighs and buttocks as, when the system is sluggish, this is where cellulite is only too likely to appear.

● Reach as much of your back as you can and then very gently massage your abdomen and chest.

● Finally, scrub your arms and shoulders, as well as your hands themselves.

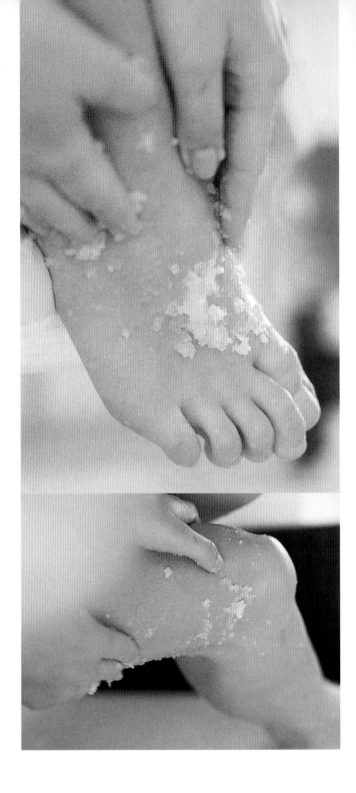

3 Step back under the shower and massage the scrub into your skin under the water until it has all been washed off. Turn the water temperature down to cold (cool, if you can't face it) and stay under the spray for a further minute, making sure that the water flows over your whole body.

● Wrap up in a warm towel and dry vigorously. Put on a warm dressing gown and lie down for five minutes. If you feel at all chilly, get back under the duvet. You should now feel a tingle all over your body.

saturday 10:00 am
salt scrub

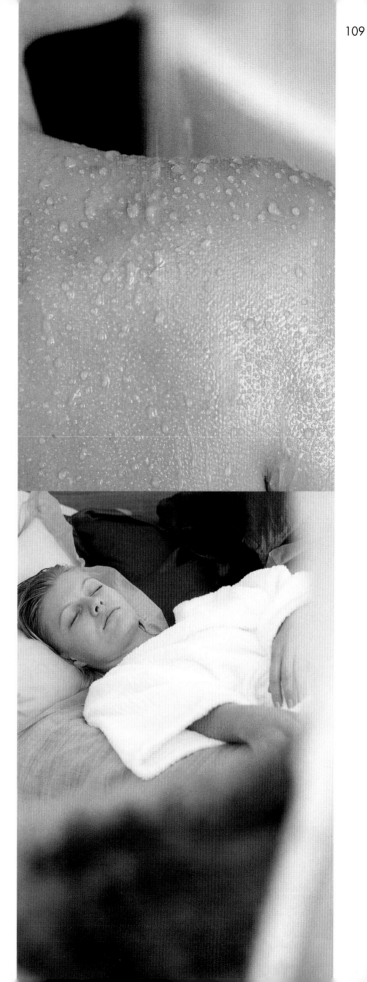

saturday 10:30 am **aromatherapy**

Many people think of aromatherapy oils as a cure for problems such as insomnia or anxiety, with an action that is fundamentally calming and tranquillizing. However, they can do quite the opposite and pep you up, too.

Following your body scrub, make up the aromatherapy body oil (see opposite). It is designed to give you a lift that will last the whole day.

You can use aromatherapy oils:
- in a vaporizer light bulb ring to scent the room.
- directly on a radiator (although this will last for less time and, obviously, only works when the radiator is on).

One of the best oils to use for this is basil, which is particularly stimulating. Others include rosemary, for a more warming, strengthening effect, peppermint, which is both invigorating and soothing, particularly if you are prone to headaches or stomach upsets, or clary sage, which is also an antidepressant. Only use one oil at a time. If you are going out, put two drops of one of these oils on a tissue or handkerchief and inhale when you feel as if you are flagging.

Caution: Do not use clary sage essential oil if you suffer from high blood pressure.

Remember that the best time of day for using all of these oils is the morning. If you use them too late in the day, the effect may be overstimulating and may even cause insomnia. If you have chronic fatigue, caused at least in part by poor sleep, have an aromatherapy bath (see pages 56–57) before you go to bed and do your final autogenic training for the day. A drop or two of lavender oil on a tissue placed on your pillow will soothe away any tension or anxiety and will help you sleep.

If you can fall asleep easily but have a problem with waking up in the night, try the self-massage on page 58–59 and put a few more drops of lavender on your pillow – neroli and marjoram are effective, too. Above all, try not to worry about lack of sleep, as this thought may keep you awake more than anything else. The combination of lavender oil and autogenic training is very successful, so just relax and let them take over.

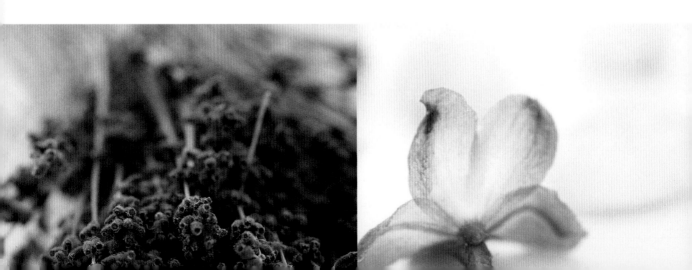

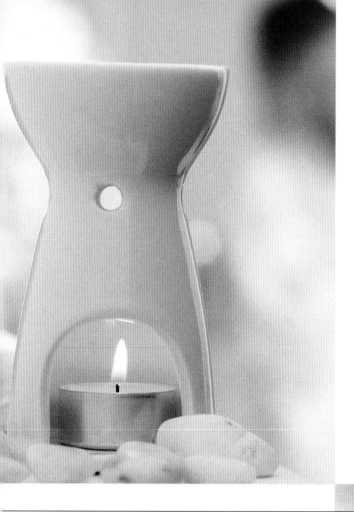

Aromatherapy body oil

- Pour 1 fl oz (25 ml) of carrier oil (grapeseed if you have normal to oily skin, olive or wheatgerm if you have dry or mature skin) into a glass bottle.
- Add to this 5 drops of lavender essential oil, 5 drops of juniper berry oil and 2 drops of cypress oil.

This is a very good mixture with which to start the day, it:
- stimulates the circulation.
- purifies the bloodstream.
- has a simultaneously calming and uplifting effect.

Massage all over your body (except your face) and keep your dressing gown on until all of it has been absorbed.

saturday 3:00 pm **ayurveda**

Ayurveda is traditional Indian medicine, the benefits of which are gradually becoming more widely recognized. One of the most simultaneously energizing and relaxing treatments is *panchakarma*, Ayurvedic massage. There are numerous different forms of *panchakarma* (PK) massage, and as more PK massage therapists are becoming trained, the massage is becoming more widespread. If you have access to a therapist, book a session as a special weekend treat.

Panchakarma treatments have been found to have remarkable effects on both mind and body. These include:
- reducing the risk factors for heart disease and infection.
- increasing strength and energy.
- improving memory, alertness and sleep patterns.

The basic massage is *abhyanga*, which means "loving hands." It usually begins with a head, face and shoulder massage. This leads on to the body massage. The most surprising features for people used to other forms of massage are that the oil used is hot sesame oil, and that you are massaged by two therapists at once. The effect is hypnotic; tensed muscles seem to become as fluid as the oil pouring over them.

Abhyanga is often followed by *shirodhara*, a treatment which does for your mind what *abhyanga* does for your body. A thin drizzle of sesame oil passes slowly back and forth across your brow, like a pendulum, pausing almost imperceptibly each time it reaches the center of the temples. *Shirodhara* lasts for 20 minutes and many people compare its effect to transcendence, the meditator's state of bliss. Other treatments include *pinda swedana*, a massage with a sort of rice pudding wrapped in muslin; *urdvartana*, a stimulating, exfoliating massage that increases circulation and promotes weight loss; and *pzzichilli*, in which literally gallons of warm oil are poured continuously over the body while it is very gently massaged for around two hours.

If you do not have access to a PK therapist, there is a certain amount you can try at home. The first thing to aim for is to get the rhythm of your day right. According to ayurveda, every day and every season has a rhythm, and the more you are attuned to it, the healthier and more energized you will feel. For example, an early bedtime is a very important part of the natural daily rhythm. So are rising early and early mealtimes. The main meal of the day should be lunch rather than supper, which should be a lighter meal.

You can try a sesame oil massage at home. If you have a

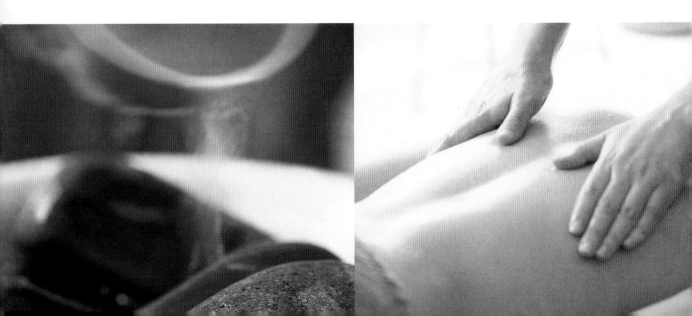

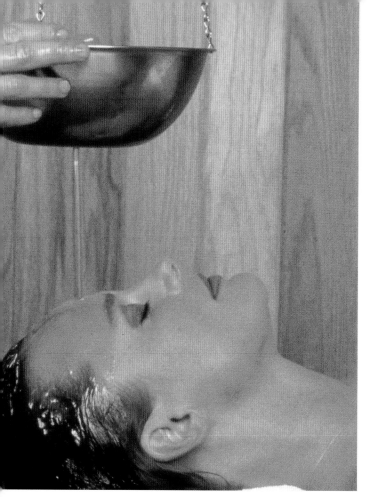

friend who is doing the Energizing Weekend with you, you could take turns to give each other a body massage (see pages 76–78). In this case, however, use sesame oil. Put a small bottle of it in hot water to heat it. The sensation on your skin should be of warmth, so it needs to heat for a while.

You can also do a self-massage. Heat the oil in the same way and then, using smooth circular movements, massage it into your whole body. Start with the soles of your feet, then work up your legs, and your body, including as much of your back as you can reach, your arms, your face, scalp and hair. Naturally, your hair will get quite oily, but you can wash it tomorrow morning. The sesame oil is very nourishing for the skin, which will be noticeably softer by tomorrow.

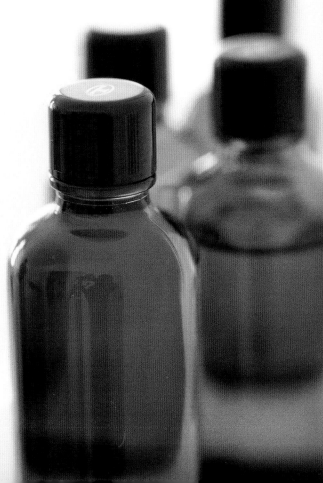

sunday

8:00 am Autogenic training	**11:00 am** Autogenic training
8:30 am Warm-up and stretches	**12:00 pm** Lunch
9:30 am High-energy drink or muesli	**3:00 pm** Chi kung
10:00 am Shower with optional salt scrub	**5:00 pm** Autogenic training
10:30 am Reflexology	**6:00 pm** Evening meal
	7:00 pm Autogenic training

Start your day with your autogenic training and exercise sessions. If you wish, you can repeat yesterday's salt scrub for the body, but not for the face, as this would be too abrasive a treatment to have two days in a row. For breakfast, choose either the yogurt drink or real muesli, with some juice and herbal tea to rehydrate your body after the night.

Take a break after breakfast. Read, listen to some music, or just relax before your next session. This is a foot massage that uses some reflexology techniques. Reflexology itself requires proper training, but some of the basic movements have been incorporated here. The underlying principle of reflexology is that there are reflex points on the feet that correspond to every organ and part of the body. The theory is that, by treating the feet, you treat the whole person.

You will find that reflexology:
- has an overall relaxing effect.
- stimulates the circulation of blood and lymph.

Many people find that even a simple foot massage makes them so relaxed they fall asleep. Clearly, this will not happen if you are massaging your own feet but if you do feel tired afterwards, lie down for half an hour before lunch.

Wear loose, comfortable clothes and sit comfortably with your back supported. You will need to find the best position to access each sole of the foot. Some people can sit cross legged with ease. Others prefer to have the foot they are massaging propped up by the other leg, which is extended in front of them. Use a firm touch throughout. Reflexology should not be practiced if you are pregnant or if you suffer from a heart condition or varicose veins.

sunday 10:30 am **reflexology**

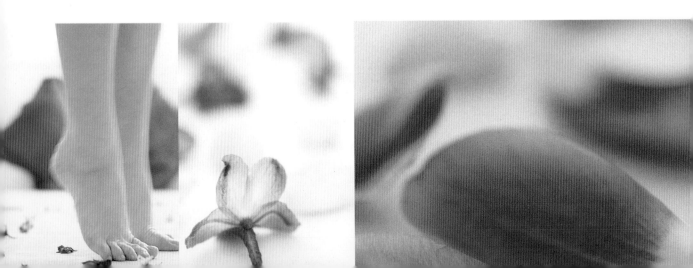

Foot massage

1 Start by relaxing your foot. Hold your foot so that one hand is on the sole and one on the top. Working from your ankle to your toes, massage it with long, firm strokes.

2 Holding your heel in one hand and your toes in the other, circle five times clockwise then counter-clockwise.

3 Starting with your big toe, stroke the length of each toe in turn and, when you reach the tip, pull gently to stretch it out. Repeat this three times.

4 Using your thumb and starting at your big toe, move along the line of pads just below your toes. Press on each one firmly before moving on to the next. Work your way to your little toe, then change hands and, using your other thumb, work your way back. Repeat twice.

5 Use your thumb to press down gently from the top to the base of your big toe. Repeat on all of your toes. When you reach your little toe, change hands and use the other thumb to go back the other way. Repeat twice.

6 Holding your toes in one hand, use your thumb on the other hand to press along the sole, pressing in a line from the base of your big toe to the center of your foot, following the line of the metatarsal. Repeat on all your toes, then repeat on the top of your foot following the same line.

7 Starting at your heel, use your thumb to press along the inside edge of your foot all the way up to your big toe. Press firmly and follow the line up over your instep. Then repeat on the outside edge of your foot, from your heel to your little toe.

8 Finally, massage the lower half of your sole, using firm pressure. Rotate your ankle, as before, both clockwise and counterclockwise. Repeat step 1, using long, firm strokes from ankle to toes. Put on a cotton sock and repeat on the other foot.

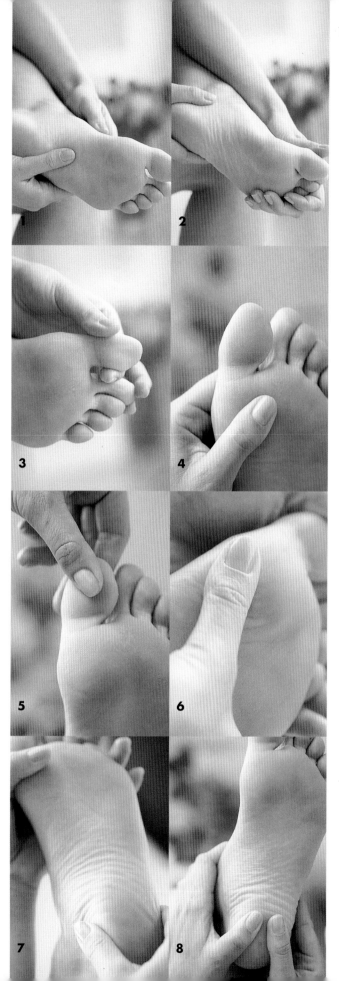

sunday 3:00 pm **chi kung**

Chi kung is a form of moving meditation and a way of harnessing and releasing the body's own vital energy, or *chi*. It can have an extraordinary beneficial effect on both physical and mental health, and it is one of the most energizing forms of exercise. There are many chi kung exercises. Some of them are for specific ailments, but the ones described here increase strength and energy, or *chi*. Given all of this, it is clearly a profound technique and one that cannot be covered in any depth in such a small amount of space. The best way to learn it is certainly to find a good teacher, go to at least one class a week and practice at home in between. Here, however, are some basic chi kung exercises to serve as an introduction to this remarkable method.

Caution: Do not do these exercises if you are pregnant.

- Dress in loose, comfortable clothing and soft shoes, socks or bare feet.

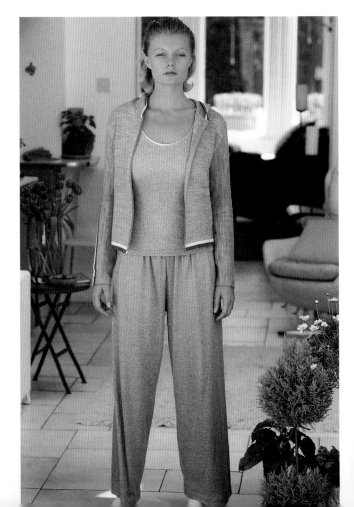

Starting position

Begin in a relaxed standing position. Make sure there is no tension in your spine. Tilt your pelvis slightly forwards to iron out your back and neck, and let your hands hang loosely at your sides. Your neck should follow the line of your spine, so your gaze is straight ahead. Relax your knees.

Lifting the sky

1 From the starting position (see opposite), bring your arms in front of your body, fingertips touching and palms facing the floor.

2 Start to raise your arms out to the sides in a wide circle.

3 When your arms are level with the top of your head, turn the palms to face the ceiling and bring them directly overhead. As far as you can, straighten your arms, with your hands at right angles to your arms, fingertips slightly apart. Hold the stretch for a moment and then lower your arms until your hands are just above your head. Raise and lower in a continuous arc up to 20 times.

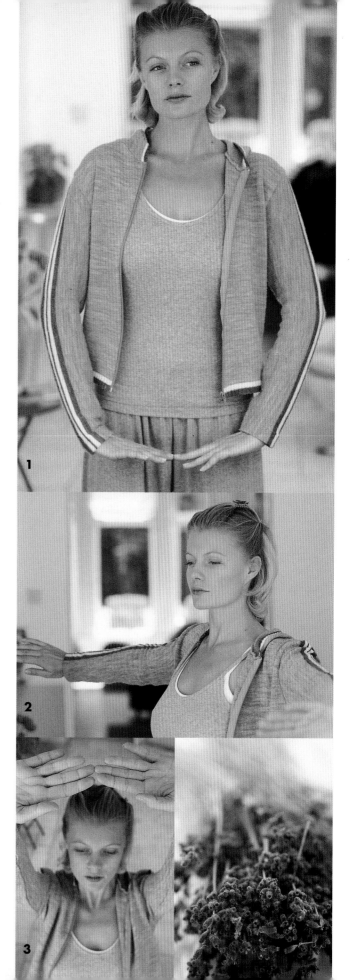

Low knee bend

1 Begin in the starting position (see page 116) and open your arms to your sides at shoulder height, palms facing upwards.

2 Breathe in and turn your palms so that they face downwards. Bring your arms up so they stretch straight out in front of you. Start to bend your knees.

3 Breathe out and bend your knees as if you were squatting or sitting on a beach ball.
● Breathe in and return to standing, with your arms still stretched in front of you.

4 Lower your arms to your sides, palms facing backwards. If you feel strong enough, repeat the sequence at least four more times.

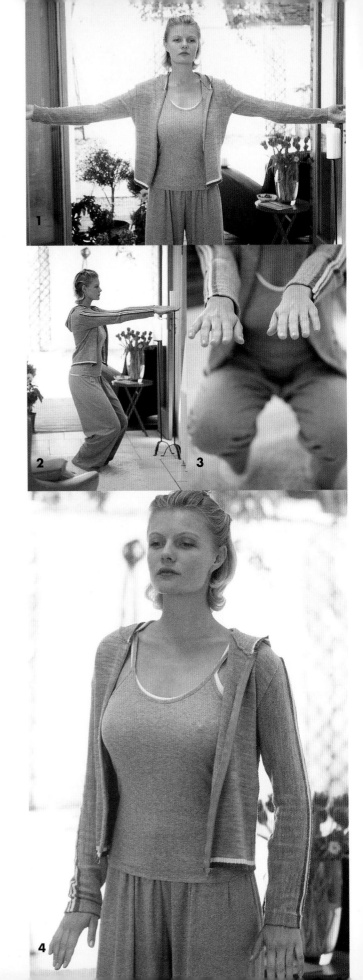

Embrace the tree

1 Stand in the starting position. Let your knees bend and feel your body's center of gravity lower, but keep your spine straight.

● Slowly raise your arms so they make a wide open circle in front of you, palms facing your chest. Stand in this position for one minute (with practice, it would be five minutes) and try to relax into it.

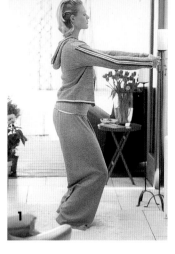

sunday 3:00 pm
chi kung

Pushing mountains

1 Stand in the starting position (see page 116). Bend your arms at the elbows, palms facing forward, drawing your arms back.

2 Push forwards from the heels of the hands. Draw the arms back again and then repeat up to 20 times.

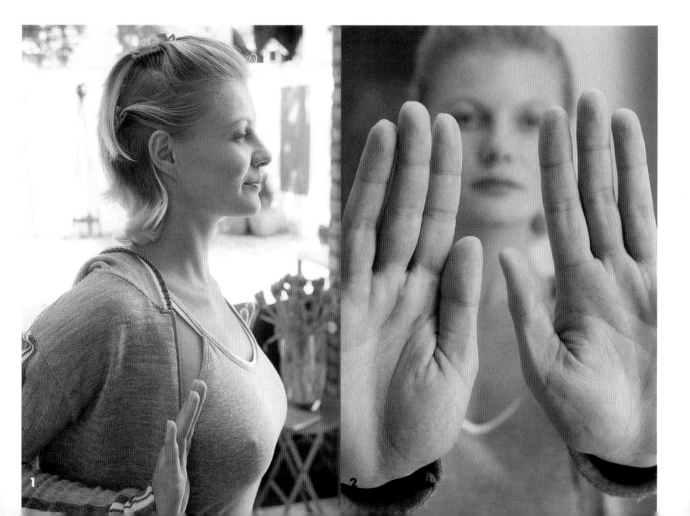

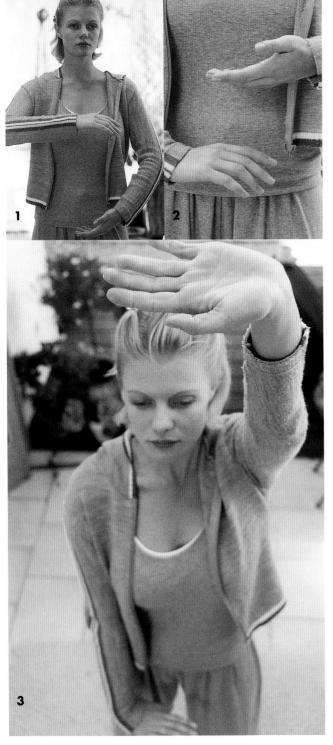

Plucking stars

1 Stand in the starting position (see page 116). Hold your arms out in front of you, elbows bent, your left arm level with your abdomen, the right at chest level, as if you were holding a beach ball.

2 Lift the left hand upwards, so the two hands pass by each other. When your left hand is level with your face, twist your arm round to allow the palm of your hand to continue to push towards the sky. The right hand should push simultaneously down towards the floor.

3 Push hard enough so that both arms straighten, fingers pointing inwards.

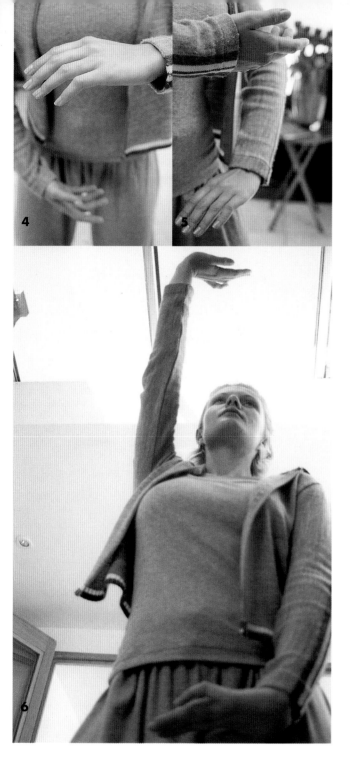

4 Reverse the arms to hold the ball again, this time with your left hand uppermost.

5 Lift the right hand upwards, turning your wrist up. Meanwhile bring your left hand down, to push towards the ground. This is the same position as step 2, but using the opposite arms.

6 Straighten both arms as in step 3.
● Repeat up to 10 times.

sunday 3:00 pm chi kung

sunday 5:00 pm **autogenic training 2**

You may feel ready to go on to stage two, or even stage three, of your autogenic training before the end of the weekend, but there should certainly be no pressure to get further than is absolutely comfortable. The main point of AT is that you relax. If you don't feel completely relaxed with the stage that you are at, don't progress. Wait until you do feel relaxed and then the next stage will give you more benefit.

If you wish, and if you feel ready, you can go on to stage 2 or stage 3 this weekend. However, this is such a useful technique that you will probably want to keep it up, so the next several stages are also outlined below. It is important to emphasize, however, that these should take weeks. Go slowly and relax.

Stage 2

When you have practiced stage 1 sufficiently and you find yourself going into relaxation very easily, go on to stage 2. Here, you lengthen the session a little by adding one further step. Repeat each phrase slowly, with pauses, as before.

- My right arm is heavy.
- My left arm is heavy.
- Both my arms are heavy.
- My right leg is heavy.
- My left leg is heavy.
- Both my legs are heavy.
- My arms and legs are heavy.
- My neck and shoulders are heavy.

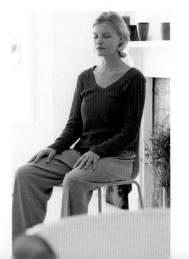

Stage 3

Now a third center for your focus is added – the breathing. This is not a particularly deep breath but, as you can see from the phrase "My body breathes me," you become aware of how the breath is affecting your entire body. Again, you repeat all of the phrases from the previous stage first.

- My right arm is heavy.
- My left arm is heavy.
- Both my arms are heavy.
- My right leg is heavy.
- My left leg is heavy.
- Both my legs are heavy.
- My arms and legs are heavy.
- My neck and shoulders are heavy.
- My body breathes me.

sunday 5:00 pm **autogenic training 2**

Stage 4

Do not attempt this stage until you can really feel the focus of the first three. Stage 3, when you add the breathing, usually takes quite a long time to focus on – so give yourself plenty of time. Here, you take your focus to your face; try to feel the sensation of coolness. When you feel ready, go on to the next stage, with the same speed, pauses and repetitions.

- My right arm is heavy.
- My left arm is heavy.
- Both my arms are heavy.
- My right leg is heavy.
- My left leg is heavy.
- Both my legs are heavy.
- My arms and legs are heavy.
- My neck and shoulders are heavy.
- My body breathes me.
- My forehead is cool and relaxed.

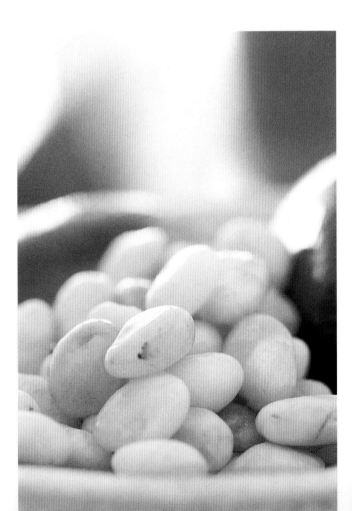

Stage 5

Again, don't rush into this stage. Here, you take your focus within to become aware of your heartbeat.

- My right arm is heavy.
- My left arm is heavy.
- Both my arms are heavy.
- My right leg is heavy.
- My left leg is heavy.
- Both my legs are heavy.
- My arms and legs are heavy.
- My neck and shoulders are heavy.
- My body breathes me.
- My forehead is cool and relaxed.
- My heartbeat is calm and regular.

Stage 6

Finally, you take your focus to the mind itself.

- My right arm is heavy.
- My left arm is heavy.
- Both my arms are heavy.
- My right leg is heavy.
- My left leg is heavy.
- Both my legs are heavy.
- My arms and legs are heavy.
- My neck and shoulders are heavy.
- My body breathes me.
- My forehead is cool and relaxed.
- My heartbeat is calm and regular.
- My mind is calm and serene.

There are other elements that can be included and you will certainly be introduced to them if you train with an AT teacher. Here, however, if you have taken it slowly enough, you will have gained enough of the essence of autogenic training for it to be of real and lasting benefit. To continue in your everyday life, do at least two sessions a day and mini-sessions if you find yourself in stressful situations.

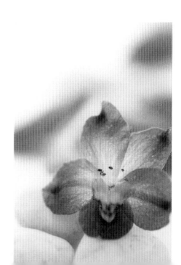

Index

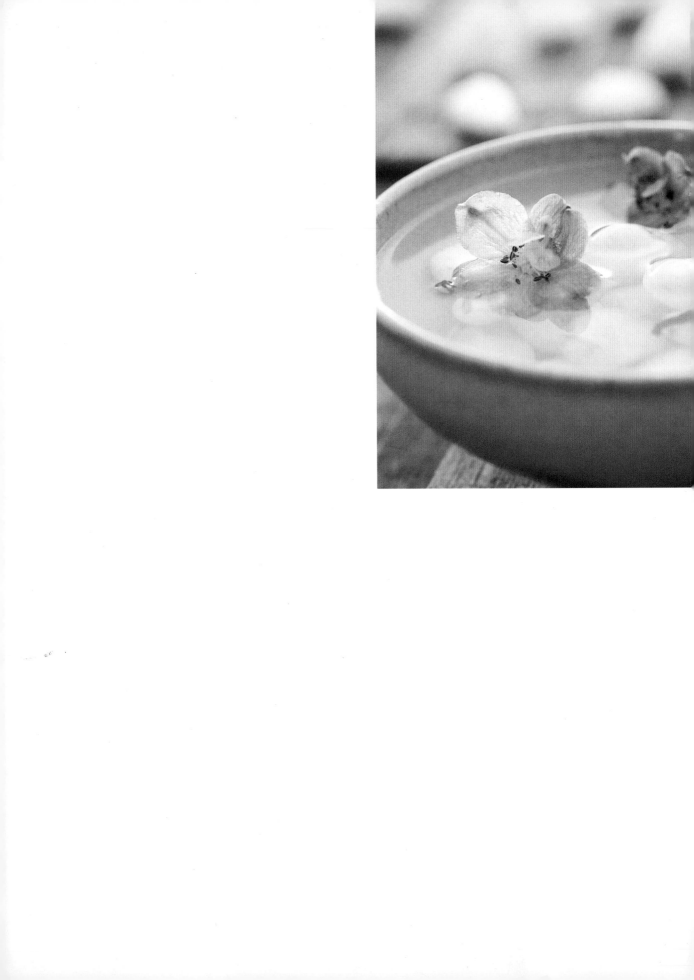